THE GP TRAINER'S

Paul Middleton

and

Steve Field

RADCLIFFE MEDICAL PRESS

© 2001 Paul Middleton and Steve Field

Radcliffe Medical Press Ltd
18 Marcham Road, Abingdon, Oxon OX14 1AA

British Library Cataloguing in Publication Data

A catalogue record for this book is available from the British Library.

ISBN 1 85775 481 6

Typeset by Advance Typesetting Ltd, Oxon
Printed and bound by TJ International Ltd, Padstow, Cornwall

► CONTENTS

3 Learning needs assessment: how do trainers assess the learning needs of registrars?   43

Introduction
Needs assessment of knowledge
Assessment of skill
Needs assessment of attitudes
Other methods for assessing needs
Summary comments

4 Teaching consultation skills: how do trainers teach consultation skills?   61

Introduction
Patient contact-related methods
Role play
Tutorial-based exercises
Assessing consultation skills and needs
Summary comments
Appendix to Chapter 4

5 Curriculum-based resources: how do trainers define a curriculum?   97

Introduction
Objectives-related methods of curriculum
    development
Process-related methods of curriculum
    development
Summary comments
Appendix to Chapter 5

6 Tutorial planning: how do trainers plan tutorials?

Introduction
Tutorial structure
Style
Theory
Feedback
Specific teaching tools
Problems of 1:1 teaching
Other points to note
Planning the tutorial – a skeleton guide
Summary comments
Appendix to Chapter 6

7 Management and change: how do trainers cover practice management issues and the concepts of management of change?

Introduction
The 'why' of management
The 'how' of management
The 'what' of management
Teams
Assertiveness
Leadership
Delegation
Other points to note
Summary comments
Appendix to Chapter 7

10 Resources: what information technology and reference sources are trainers using?   281

Introduction
References – for registrars
References – for trainers
Other resources
Summary comments

11 The written word: what books do trainers recommend? What other sources of information do trainers use?   293

Introduction
General advice
Books
Information technology (IT)
The practice library
Summary comments
Appendix to Chapter 11

12 Troubleshooting: how do trainers deal with the 'difficult' registrar?   319

Introduction
The problems
Approaches
Summary comments

► ACKNOWLEDGEMENTS

This handbook is a collective effort with many contributors. The 100 trainers who put pen to paper are listed on pp. xi–xiii: without their efforts this handbook would not have been possible. I am very grateful to all of them.

I also owe a debt of gratitude to Dr Guan Yeo and the staff of the North Ryde, NSW, RACGP training programme. Not only did the Australian spring help produce an environment for these ideas to bud, but the staff at North Ryde fertilised the process wonderfully.

I would also like to thank Dr Carl Whiteside and everyone at the Faculty of Family Medicine, University of British Columbia, Vancouver, who helped the bud develop in the beautiful colours of the Canadian fall.

The project would not have been possible without tremendous support from Dr Steve Field and his staff at the West Midlands Regional Department of Postgraduate General Practice Training.

I am grateful for encouragement from the Royal College of General Practitioners and in particular to Dr David Haslam for his comments. I would also like to thank the NHS Executive for financial support for my prolonged study leave and Allen and Hanburys for their contribution towards the computing requirements.

Finally I would like to encourage my fellow trainers out there in the front line of the training world to speak up and spread their ideas so we can all share the gems of GP education.

Paul Middleton
September 2000

I am very grateful to Paul for asking me to become involved in his 'big project'. It was Paul who came to me with a brilliant idea for his Prolonged Study Leave and subsequently drove the project forward. Paul has moved on from being a trainer to being one of the West Midlands' most dynamic and visionary Course Organisers. The experience that he gained in his travels to Australia and Canada have enriched vocational training schemes across the Region.

The experience gained chairing the implementation group for the UK GP Registrar Training Scheme has helped me in the development of this book. I, therefore, thank all of the members of the group for their help and support over the last two years.

My final thank you is to add to Paul's acknowledgement of the input of the hundred or so West Midlands Trainers. They have been and continue to be innovative, challenging, creative and above all very supportive – I am very grateful for their help!

Steve Field
September 2000

► ABOUT THE AUTHORS

Paul Middleton joined his rural general practice on the Welsh border in 1987 after six years as a RAF Medical Officer. He started as a GP Trainer in 1989 and rapidly became aware of the tremendous support and inspiration that his fellow Trainers provided. His interest in training was broadened by his experience as an MRCGP examiner from 1993. This reinforced the belief that sharing peer group experience produced a major enhancement in the learning process of the GP Trainer.

Paul continues to train and examine for the MRCGP and summative assessment and has recently become a Vocational Training Scheme Course Organiser in Shropshire. His enthusiasm for the training process is still constantly enriched by his colleagues and learners.

Steve Field has been a GP since 1986 in both rural Worcestershire and inner city Birmingham. His previous experience has involved running the Worcestershire Vocational Training Scheme and starting the West Midlands Modular Trainers Course which opened up the possibility of becoming a GP Trainer to more women in the West Midlands. He is currently Director of Post-graduate GP Education for the West Midlands and Vice Chairman of the Committee of General Practice Education Directors (CoGPED). In his spare time he is also Chairman of the Guidance Implementation Group which introduced the new GP Registrar Scheme across the United Kingdom in April 2000!

Steve is committed to the development of high-quality education and training for general practice so that the GPs of the future will have the appropriate skills, knowledge and competencies necessary to meet the needs of their NHS patients. One of his most formative experiences was attending the Foundation Trainers Course at Keele University, which showed him the need for good quality courses and support for young trainers. This book is part of his mission to support GP Trainers both in the West Midlands and across the United Kingdom.

THE '100 TRAINERS GUIDE TO TRAINING': THE CONTRIBUTORS

Dr S Adams, Hereford
Dr M Allen, Northfield
Dr P Barritt, Shrewsbury
Dr J Bartlett, Wem
Dr J Bennett, Clive
Dr J Blacker, Bromsgrove
Dr F Borchardt, Pershore
Dr T Breese, Oswestry
Dr J Brown, Lichfield
Dr S Brown, Brinklow
Dr S Brown, Stirchley
Dr M Camm, Balsall Common
Dr A Canale-Parola, Rugby
Dr G Carpenter, Leek
Dr C Cheel, Bartley Green
Dr S Clay, Erdington
Dr S Collier, Warley
Dr R Cherry, Bartley Green
Dr P Clayton, Ross-on-Wye
Dr G Cooper, Redditch
Dr A Coward, King's Norton
Dr G Crampton, West Bromwich
Dr T Crossley, Wolverhampton
Dr D Davies, Hereford
Dr G Davies, Clive
Dr R Davies, Kenilworth
Dr A De Cothi, Kidderminster
Dr M Deighan, Worcester

Dr J Divall, Sutton Coldfield
Dr S Edmunds, Pontesbury
Dr R Evans, Birmingham
Dr A Eyre, Hereford
Dr S Gabriel, Birmingham
Dr T Gasper, Stratford-on-Avon
Dr P Glennon, Stafford
Dr P Griffiths, Birmingham
Dr S Hallatt, Shrewsbury
Dr C Halpin, Tamworth
Dr W Hammerton, Bridgnorth
Dr J Hardwick, Kidderminster
Dr K Harrison, Walsall
Dr R Hayward, Newcastle-under-Lyme
Dr B Herriot, Malvern
Dr R Holzman, Kidderminster
Dr R Horton, Burton-on-Trent
Dr A Houghton, Stretton-on-Dunsmore
Dr D Hughes, Leek
Dr P Gupta, Dudley
Dr J Hagon, Solihull
Dr A Jaron, Smethwick
Dr R Jenkins, Bromsgrove
Dr M Jones, Stafford
Dr F Kameen, Droitwich
Dr K Keohane, Telford
Dr K King, Stratford-on-Avon
Dr A Leeman, Ross-on-Wye
Dr D Lowden, Baschurch
Dr G Luckraft, Wolverhampton
Dr Y Lydon, Tutbury
Dr J McDonnell, Birmingham
Dr P Middleton, Oswestry
Dr M Mortimer, Smethwick
Dr P Moszuti, Walsall
Dr D Munslow, Stafford
Dr W Norton, Barbourne
Dr H Nutbeam, Warley

Dr D O'Brien, Hereford
Dr A Otter, Shrewsbury
Dr G Paige, Coventry
Dr S Parnell, Kingswinford
Dr O Penny, Weobley
Dr M Perry, Albrighton
Dr S Powell, Newport
Dr W Price, Warley
Dr C Prince, Bewdley
Dr Pryke, Bromsgrove
Dr D Rapley, Kenilworth
Dr D Rivers, Warwick
Dr A Robinson, Kingswinford
Dr K Robinson, Church Stretton
Dr P Robinson, Bidford-on-Avon
Dr J Sainsbury, Cannock
Dr A Seeley, Bridgnorth
Dr J Siegel, Burton-on-Trent
Dr J Sihota, Coventry
Dr R Spencer-Jones, Tutbury
Dr T Stenhouse, Solihull
Dr I Stuart, Solihull
Dr I Sykes, Tividale
Dr C Taggart, Coventry
Dr E Tattersall, Sudbury
Dr D Towers, Smethwick
Dr I Walton, Dudley
Dr M Waters, Hereford
Dr S Watts, Solihull
Dr R Wilcox, King's Norton
Dr G Willis, Ellesmere
Dr J Woodward, Kineton

and two anonymous contributors.

My sincere apologies if I have missed any names.

► INTRODUCTION

One hundred trainers in the West Midlands completed an in-depth questionnaire about their educational methods and philosophy of training. This handbook is the product of their efforts. The handbook is a 'bottom-up' approach to education: it describes the practicalities of training, and offers solutions to problems and thoughts on training from a large number of people who train registrars from day to day.

Individual trainers develop their own style and techniques: some modified from other sources, others personally crafted: these are the gems of GP postgraduate education. These gems are dug out of the mine of experience, information, paperwork, books and advice that bombard the trainer. The handbook is a collection of some of these gems. Some of them are polished and sophisticated, others are the uncut stones. The reader is left to make the setting and test out their value.

What are trainers trying to achieve in postgraduate GP training? This is a question trainers must keep at the forefront of their minds when training. This handbook is a treasure chest of techniques that may, or may not, be helpful in particular training situations. Many trainers would rightly say that it is outcome and not process we are ultimately concerned about. However, it seems a valid assumption that a varied, stimulating and multi-faceted approach to training is likely to be beneficial for both trainer and registrar.

Paul Middleton
Steve Field
September 2000

INTRODUCTION

► HOW TO USE THIS HANDBOOK

This handbook contains many practical tools, resource ideas, interesting theories (some even useful!), and advice to help new and established trainers. It is not designed to be a programme for training. It is designed to disseminate a range of ideas and options that many trainers use regularly.

Trainers can use it in a number of ways:

- ► to stimulate thought in a particular area of training
- ► to look for options in particular training areas
- ► to find resource material in particular areas
- ► to act as an overview of the training process.

The contents pages enable identification of the relevant chapter and section.

Most of the chapters mention sources of advice or practical help. Wherever possible, the appendix to the chapter will contain the material required or details of how to acquire it. The details provided are as complete as possible – in some rare instances (i.e. material currently out of print) more established trainers in your area may be able to help.

Some chapters simply describe what trainers felt were the key elements of an area. This can form the basis for tutorial construction.

All the chapters have margins for notes: the handbook is a practical tool and each trainer using the tools will have his or her own views on how well they work. The margin is for your comments and modifications. Where there is a significant degree of overlap between chapters the essentials points have been reiterated.

We hope this handbook will prove a useful addition to the trainer's 'toolbox'. Its central message is the philosophy of learning by and sharing of experience. So remember: tell as many trainers as possible about your own 'gems'.

CHAPTER 1

Induction to practice: how do trainers settle registrars into their practices?

'Sit down and have some tea' said the Mad Hatter

Lewis Carroll (*Alice in Wonderland*)

Introduction

I can remember feeling just like Alice at the Mad Hatter's party when I arrived in general practice. Here I was, after years of training, raring to go. But patients kept describing things that baffled me, and that was when they *were* ill – most of them hadn't even got the good grace to have an illness at all! I was either mad or the rules had changed – like Alice I discovered the latter was true.
Paul Middleton

Sadly this still appears to be true to a degree today.

So what do trainers do about it? Maslow's hierarchy of human needs is one method of looking at this problem. Neighbour in the *Inner Apprentice* develops this concept into the hierarchy of educational perspectives. These hierarchies are shown in Boxes 1.1 and 1.2.

Box 1.1: Maslow's hierarchy of human needs

Self-actualisation
realisation of innate potential
self-expression
self-fulfilment
self-respect
self-confidence

Esteem needs
esteem
status
approval

Belongingness needs
love
intimacy
acknowledgement

Safety needs
boundaries
predictability
stability

Physiological needs
sleep
sex
food/drink, etc.

Box 1.2: Hierarchy of educational needs

Autonomy
takes responsibility for own learning
successfully evolves from registrar to principal
sense of purpose, worth and direction

Self-esteem
uses self in consultation
achieves a balanced lifestyle
tolerates uncertainty, occasional mistakes
knows limitations
can challenge accepted wisdom/trainer

Recognition
hungry for new ideas
interested in the wider sphere of primary care
can accept praise/criticism
confidence growing independent of trainer

Confidence
accepted in primary healthcare team
uses and contributes to primary healthcare team
bonds with trainer
sees wider scope of spectrum of illness

Safety
able and willing to ask for help
knows where to access resources
basic clinical skills and knowledge

Survival
knows timetable
satisfactory environment
working knowledge of admin systems (phones, paperwork,
geography, services, etc.)
free enough from non-medical worries

These lists can be used to develop an introductory programme that allows registrars to feel their way into general practice. Maslow's scale is now considered flawed (when did you last get out of bed because your self-esteem was calling? And what does 'self-actualisation' actually mean? The answer being that if you have to ask you don't have it!). Figure 1.1 (from Glasser 1965) illustrates a more accepted model of human needs based on survival (i.e. you actually got out of bed to survive and this figure illustrates your survival drives, and no self-actualisation either!).

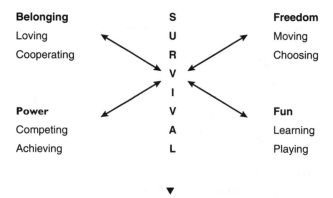

Figure 1.1: Glasser's motivating factors.

These models provide food for thought when trying to introduce the new registrar to the practice – all trainers have to do is make them feel happy, stimulated and clever, free and loved – it's that simple!

That's enough preamble – what about some practical points?

The appointment of GP registrars

In March 2000, the Minister of Health, Lord Hunt, launched a new UK guide to the GP registrar scheme. The launch heralded a profound change in the funding arrangements for vocational training and brought with it opportunity for new flexible approaches to GP training. Under the new arrangements, funding for GP vocational training has been transferred from the General Medical Services budget to the Medical Dental Education Levy (MADEL) – for this reason the change is also known as the MADEL transfer. The change followed an historic agreement between the Department of Health and the General Practitioners Committee at the BMA in 1999. The funds transferred relate to all aspects of GP training which was originally described in Chapter 38 of the Statement of Fees and Allowances (the Red Book). The details of the regulations differ across the UK but the principle is the same. From April 2000, recruitment to vocational training schemes and to general practice training placements is the responsibility of the Directors of Postgraduate General Education (DsPGPE).

The DsPGPE aim to ensure that the recruitment process is open and based fairly on the principle of equal opportunities for all applicants. Part-time, flexible training and doctors wishing to return to general practice are also actively encouraged. The DsPGPE are each working on new systems of recruitment, which differ slightly between each deanery. The aim is that by working together they will develop a centralised system similar to the UCAS system for recruiting students to universities. While the development work continues in the individual deaneries, the common theme is that GP registrars will be placed in a general practice with the agreement of trainers rather than the old system whereby GP trainers would advertise and select potential registrars themselves. The old system was open to many accusations of sexism and racism. The new system should avoid all of that.

The advertising and recruitment for all posts will be synchronised across the UK. National advertisements will be placed twice a year in the *British Medical Journal*, on the Department of Health website and other websites such as www.primarycareonline.co.uk. The interview and selection process will be managed by the deanery, and once selected for training the registrar will then be invited to choose a practice. The exact method of how registrars choose their practices varies from deanery to deanery. In some deaneries a matching plan is being used, in others it is left for the registrar and the trainers to make their own arrangements.

Because of the flexibility under the MADEL transfer arrangements it will be increasingly common for registrars to be offered extensions to their training year to allow them to fulfil their personal learning needs. There are also increasing training opportunities, in a general practice setting, for learning more about women's health, diabetes, mental illness, and even exposure to what it is like to work in an inner city area.

The registrars appointed by the deanery will have been selected in an open system based on the best principles of equal opportunities. The trainer will continue to enter into an employment contract with the registrar and will therefore wish to meet the registrar, review their curriculum vitae, and check their references, GMC and Medical Defence certificates. They will be supported by the paperwork supplied by the deanery.

What do trainers put in introductory booklets?

These booklets are a common tool and usually contain a lot of useful information. The following list can be used as a checklist to consider inclusions. It also acts as a reminder of the areas to cover with new registrars, even if not formally put in writing:

- an index
- an introduction to the booklet, stressing where to get help and DON'T PANIC

- a brief practice profile (numbers of patients, characteristics of area, major health needs, pattern of service provision, social activities, etc.)
- a timetable. This should give details of surgery times, tutorial and half-day commitments, on-call arrangements and particularly details of cover for each activity
- an introduction to the staff (names, job titles, who to ask what, staff structure, etc.)
- an introduction to the clinical staff: doctors, nurses, etc. (names, qualifications, interests, addresses, etc.)
- geographical data (maps, street maps, etc.)
- a 'need-to-know' list (*see* Appendix to Chapter 5) prioritising what to try and pick up quickly. Registrars often feel flooded at the start
- a list of telephone numbers (*see* example list in the appendix to this chapter)
- a list of the potential outside visits (*see* example in the appendix to this chapter)
- the 'difficult' list (*see* 'The 'difficult' list' section in Chapter 5)
- a statement of educational philosophy, i.e. why you train
- a statement of the registrar's rights and responsibilities with regard to training. The example in the Appendix to this chapter arose out a joint registrar/trainer study day
- practice leaflet
- the initial needs assessment package (*see* Chapter 3)
- the relevant regional documentation (*see* Chapter 2)
- the contract for the registrar (*see* Chapter 2)
- sometimes a job description for the registrar
- brief notes on the referral process (i.e. where, who, etc.)
- a list of available equipment, i.e. auroscope, ophthalmoscope, tendon hammer, tuning fork, stethoscope, fluoroscein, eye loup, visual acuity charts, peak flow meter, dermatome chart, asthma inhalers for demonstration, weight scales and height measure, tongue depressor, sonicaid, urinalysis sticks, glucometer, speculum, etc.

- other available equipment in the surgery, e.g. audiometry, proctoscope, spirometer, sigmoidoscope, arterial doppler, 24-hour BP monitor, pregnancy tests, cautery, cryocautery, curette, autoclave, centrifuge, microscope, resuscitation equipment
- a library and IT use advice guide
- an introductory timetable and weekly timetable
- an introduction to the day release course
- an introduction to summative assessment/MRCGP
- an introduction to the use of video (*see* Chapter 9)
- administrative/financial advice on the vagaries of the red book, etc.
- advice on relevant practice policies/procedures, i.e. venepuncture, minor surgery, chaperones, communication within the primary healthcare team (PHCT), result notification system, visit and telephone contact systems, mail systems and clinical protocols where appropriate
- a list of dates to cover deanery/regional courses, half-day releases, summative assessment deadlines, etc.
- a reminder of the requirements necessary for child health, family planning, minor surgery and obstetric list approval
- other (articles on doctors' bag, etc.; *see* 'References – for registrars' section in Chapter 10).

This is a daunting list – for both registrar and trainer. However, once written, the booklet is easy to keep up to date. As long as it is treated as a reference manual and not a tome for rote learning then the feedback from registrars is usually good. A nice addition is a section for the outgoing registrars to add any useful comments for the next incumbent.

What do trainers plan in an induction course?

Many practices plan a specific 1–2-week induction course for registrars. This usually involves the following.

Structural components

▸ Joint surgeries and visits with many partners

Comment: this allows the registrar to develop the 'belonging' concept, pick up many of the practical tips and begin to appreciate different consultation styles. There is the potential for this 'Sitting with Nellie' to lose value and it sometimes helps to prime the registrar with a filter, i.e. attempt to focus his or her attention without being too directive. This can be pre-written in his or her diary or done as a sort of prompt card (*see* Box 1.3).

Box 1.3: Prompt card example

Prompt card for joint surgery with partner A

'Every doctor is the best doctor in the world at one thing – but they don't know what it is! Can you find it? And learn it?'
'What does partner A do well? How could you learn this?'
'What does partner A do that surprises you? Why does it surprise you? Did you ask why he did this?'

▸ Joint surgeries with other PHCT members

Comment: this usually means the practice nurse, health visitor, physiotherapist, district nurse and social worker.

Extending this to a session in appointments or taking visit requests, visiting a chemist or even just sitting in the waiting room for an hour can be useful. It helps the registrar if he or she can consider what he or she should learn from each of these sessions, with filters if necessary, and to consider if the PHCT member involved requires any training in teaching techniques.

▶ Session with administrator

Comment: the actual person to do this may vary but the content needs to cover the essentials of salary, allowances (relocation, telephone, car, etc.), professional details (hopefully already checked, i.e. medical defence, GMC certificate) and other administrative detail (phone numbers, addresses, accommodation, on-call details, surgery alarm numbers, relevant keys).

▶ Deanery paperwork

Comment: most deaneries bombard the registrar with booklets on summative assessment and induction courses. Sometimes it seems weeks before the registrar is allowed to feel it is time to settle into the practice. A warning that many feel like this can help.

▶ Tutorials

Comment: the first few tutorials usually cover the 'essentials' whatever *they* are! In practice they seem to cover:

– prescription forms
– essential practice systems
– basic computer use
– common presentations
– contraception
– the ill child
– the PHCT
– sick notes.

Process elements

▶ Educational philosophy

Comment: in order to foster the learning environment this is the time to start the role modelling process. It is also the time to introduce motivating processes (fun, competition, belongingness, freedom). The registrar should have a stimulating, enjoyable, challenging and personally rewarding introduction. Doesn't that sound easy within a busy practice!

▶ Video

Comment: you can never start early enough with this – the technicalities (*see* Chapter 9), practicalities and philosophy (*see* Chapter 4) should be addressed in this period.

▶ Summative assessment

Comment: this needs to be started early. Chapter 8 covers this area.

▶ Formative assessment

Comment: it is helpful to emphasise the difference between formative and summative assessment at this early stage. It de-threatens the process and opens up the positive aspects of assessment that are alien to many registrars.

Summary comments

Registrars need an induction into general practice. This is probably the one area that can be standardised for most registrars. It serves as a secure basis on which to build. It allows both the registrar and the trainer time to settle in, time to plan and time to allow the educational process to develop. The concept of role-modelling appears to be an essential element of professional education and this period provides the ideal opportunity to show the new registrar a variety of good role models. After all this perhaps the registrar and trainer should take the Mad Hatter's advice – sit down and have a cup of tea!

Appendix to Chapter 1

Educational philosophy

A statement of the rights and responsibilities of registrars

In addition to the employment contract that is signed between the trainer and the registrar, it is good practice to also have an educational contract. There is no national model for the educational contract but the example below illustrates many elements of what it should contain. It was developed by a workshop of trainers and registrars in the West Midlands Region. The registrars felt that it would be helpful to make an explicit educational agreement with the trainer at the beginning of their training year. It should be included in the introductory booklet.

The first element should contain your own 'mission statement', which makes it sound like you are heading where no man has been before (and hopefully you're not). This is a declaration of why you train. A simple one liner should do, e.g. 'This practice trains for the stimulus it provides and the satisfaction we get from helping the next generation of doctors'. Hopefully the process of the whole practice deciding on your one liner is where the benefit lies. Try it!

Sample educational contract

Educational philosophy

Why do we train? Our 'mission statement' summarises this:

....

This document tries to clarify some of the issues surrounding the learning process.

Teaching time

We aim to provide X hours face-to-face teaching tutorial time per week. This should ALWAYS happen, barring very unusual circumstances. We put a lot of effort into this time and it will be more effective if:

- an educational diary is kept by the registrar
- the registrar feels free to influence the format and content
- the registrar prepares for tutorials.

The registrar should be aware of cover from a named partner at all times and should not have any hesitation asking for advice.

Study leave

We encourage all registrars to take the full entitlement of 30 days study leave per year. X of these involve the half-day release course which we consider an essential part of your training. There are also a number of deanery study days – discuss these with your peers and the trainer. The introductory courses also take up some of this time. Thirty days is not a lot – plan your use of these carefully, bearing in mind your educational needs. Also remember the needs of the minor surgery, child health surveillance and family planning regulations, and the demands of examinations. If you feel you need more study leave discuss this with your trainer.

When you are planning study leave make sure it is appropriate within the practice. Almost always it will be, but you are now in a team and cannot assume you won't be missed.

Commitment

We believe we are an enthusiastic, well-organised practice providing good-quality care – at least most of the time! This requires commitment and we would expect the registrar to join with us in that philosophy – particularly in terms of timekeeping and communication with all of the PHCT.

Workload

The absolute rule is that a registrar will not be asked to do more than any partner. Usually it will be considerably less. The educational process is more important than the service commitment, although the latter is significant and at times may be crucial. Towards the end of the year, registrars should expect to sample the 'real' world, with a workload similar to that of a partner.

Exchanges

If you would like to arrange a practice exchange for a week or so, ask – the answer will usually be yes.

The future

An essential part of our philosophy is the desire to improve what we do. The registrar can help here by feedback to us all. We love to hear about what we do well but we are also keen to know where we can do better – if you tell us then the next patient or registrar will benefit. Please speak up.

ABOVE ALL WE GENERALLY ENJOY WHAT WE DO – SO SMILE!

Potential visits

Increasingly the members of our PHCT are practice-based and you will see them at work – but not all of them. The support and services network outside the practice is vast. Many established GPs wish they had a greater appreciation of this network. The registrar year is a fantastic opportunity to go and see some of these agencies at work. If you do want to explore this area then please discuss it with your trainer. The following list is offered as food for thought:

- social worker
- alcohol counselling service
- community psychiatric nurse (CPN)
- complementary medical practitioner
- optician
- local factory
- chemist
- coroner's court
- undertaker
- appliance fitter
- solicitor
- hospice
- ambulance service
- Macmillan nurse
- Samaritans
- job centre
- fire service
- day hospital
- police service
- outpatient clinics
- disability employment adviser
- orthoptist
- regional medical officer
- audiometrist
- Alcoholics Anonymous (AA) meeting
- physiotherapist

- ▸ community child health clinic
- ▸ chiropodist
- ▸ health authority
- ▸ dietician
- ▸ local medical committee meeting
- ▸ MAAG
- ▸ PCG/PCT Board
- ▸ PCG/PCT clinical governance lead.

Useful telephone numbers

This form is designed to be filled in with the relevant numbers you may need as a registrar.

Partners at home: ....

....

....

....

....

Practice manager at home: ....

Practice:
  Appointments: ....
  Visits: ....
  Practice manager: ....
  Prescriptions: ....
  Other: ....
  Fax: ....
  E-mail: ....

On-call related:
  Bleep: ....
  Cooperative number 1,
    for patients: ....
  Cooperative number 2,
    for doctors: ....
  Mobile phone: ....

Hospitals: ....

....

....

Health authority: ....
Course organiser: ....

Regional advisor: ....

Ambulance control: ....

Police: ....

Fire service: ....

Undertakers: ....

Coroner's officer: ....

Duty social worker: ....
    (out-of-hours)

CPN: ....

Social services: ....
    (in-hours)

Chemists: ....

Citizens' advice bureau: ....

Day hospital: ....

Physiotherapy: ....

Macmillan nurse: ....

Hospice: ....

Health visitor: ....

District nurse 1: ....
    (in-hours)

District nurse 2: ....
    (night nurse)

Opticians: ....

MAAG: ....

► CHAPTER 2

The bare essentials: what must a trainer have access to?

They're just the bear necessities of life

Baloo in *The Jungle Book* by Rudyard Kipling

Introduction

There is a theory that Western civilisation will be buried and fossilised beneath its own paperwork mountains. Many trainers would understand this concept all too well. This section aims to identify the bare essentials that a new or existing trainer should consider in terms of paperwork and other resources.

What is a GP trainer?

A GP trainer is a doctor approved by the Joint Committee on Postgraduate Training for General Practice (JCPTGP) in accordance with regulation 7 of the vocational training regulations for the purposes of training GP registrars in general practice.

To become a GP trainer a doctor must be fully registered with the General Medical Council and then be approved as a trainer by the JCPTGP. The JCPTGP makes its decision based on evidence submitted to it by the Director of Postgraduate GP Education in the area where the GP works. The vocational training regulations are quite strict. They state that the Joint Committee must be satisfied that the characteristics and qualities of both the potential trainer and the trainee practice are such that the experience required by the regular GP regulations can be provided. The JCPTGP publishes detailed guidance about the requirements for approval as a trainer. The DsPGPE appoint trainers in their deaneries, advised by their Deanery GP Education Committees.

The approval process

Although it is often the individual doctor who considers becoming a trainer, the decision involves the whole practice. Training is often a rewarding experience but it does have costs in time and effort, and occasionally it can be a source of stress within the practice. We have never met a single trainer who manages without some loss of personal time and space. It is extremely helpful to clarify the following points with all the doctors in the practice:

- Why are we considering training? Challenge, money, pair of hands, etc.?
- Are we all prepared to contribute to the process in some way? How?
- Do we all appreciate the commitment required by the trainer (time, effort, emotional costs, etc.)? Particularly commitment to workshop sessions, training days, weekly protected time for tutorials, etc.
- Are we prepared for the hidden financial costs of training (video camera, television, lost item of service payments, organisational costs, etc.)?
- How do we all feel about having another doctor in the practice, seeing our patients, challenging our views, changing our treatments, etc.?

Deaneries can establish their own criteria for the selection of trainers to reflect local circumstances and interests but these must be congruent with the recommendations of the JCPTGP laid down in their guidelines, *Recommendations to the Deaneries on the Selection of General Practice Trainers*. Training practices must meet the JCPTGP list of minimum criteria. These criteria are changed from time to time to take account of various major changes, e.g. assessments. The minimum standards published as a JCPTGP policy statement are as follows.

Quality standards

1 All medical records and hospital correspondence must be filed in the practice notes, in date order.
2 Appropriate medical records must contain easily discernible drug therapy lists for patients on long-term therapy.

3 (i) Deaneries should set and publish targets for the achievement of summaries in medical records in teaching practices.
  (ii) Practices should be seen to be making progress towards reaching these targets.
  (iii) Slow progress in an otherwise satisfactory practice should lead to a shorter period of reselection than the deanery norm.
  (iv) Joint Committee visitors will expect to receive the deanery's policy statements on summaries in medical records and will review and report on progress towards implementing this policy.

4 All training practices should have methods for monitoring prescribing habits as an important part of the audit process. They should have either a practice formulary or a prescribing list and a policy on how the list is reviewed and implemented.

5 All training practices should have a library that conforms to a recommended deanery reading list and contains a selection of books and journals relevant to general practice.

6 All training practices must provide opportunities for GP registrars to become familiar with the principles of medical audit and to participate in medical audit; they must be able to demonstrate that GP registrars have participated in medical audit.

7 All training practices must possess video cameras, which should be of sufficient technical quality to be suitable for national assessment. Trainers should work with the GP registrars to familiarise them with the use of this equipment.

8 Formative assessment, that is assessment for education purposes, should form an essential part of the training of all GP registrars.

9 Deaneries are expected to ensure that their trainers are well placed to facilitate the technical and administrative aspects of summative assessment and are aware of the appropriate sections of the Vocational Training Summative Assessment Board's *Protocol for the Management of Summative Assessment*. Following acceptance of the MRCGP's assessment of consulting skills by videotape, trainees should also be aware of the current MRCGP regulations.

10 The Joint Committee also expects all trainers and training practices to diligently observe and teach the professional guidance contained within the GMC publications *Good Medical Practice* and *Maintaining Good Medical Practice*.

Trainer selection procedures

All trainers must be formally appointed and must be subject to reselection. Doctors who wish to become trainers should apply to the Director of Postgraduate GP Education who will make arrangements for the practice to be visited. In some deaneries the prospective trainer also has to attend a trainer selection interview. The visiting team varies in composition from deanery to deanery but usually includes an associate director, a local GP trainer and/or a course organiser. In many deaneries visiting teams are becoming more multi-professional in composition; practice managers are commonly members of the team.

The form of the visit also varies between deaneries. The length of the visit may vary between three hours and a whole day, the purpose being to ensure that the doctor and the training practice achieve the deanery's and therefore the JCPTGP's standards. The deaneries also consider the following general characteristics of the doctor and the practice.

1 The attributes of the trainer as a doctor will include:

- a high standard of professional and personal values in relation to patient care
- appropriate availability and accessibility to patients
- a high standard of clinical competence
- the ability to communicate effectively
- a commitment to personal, professional development as a clinician
- a commitment to audit and peer review
- a sensitivity to the personal needs and feelings of colleagues.

2 The qualities of the trainer as a teacher will include:

- a personal commitment to teaching and learning
- an understanding of the principles and theory of education applied to medicine

- practical teaching skills
- a willingness to develop further as a clinical teacher
- a commitment to audit and peer review related to teaching
- the ability to use formative assessment and construct educational plans
- the ability to facilitate the summative assessment process.

3   A practice suitable for training will include:

- partners and staff who practice a high standard of medicine, and who are committed to vocational training
- good quality practice premises
- an effective primary care team
- involvement in quality assurance
- well organised practice records and registers or their computerised equivalents
- an appropriate level of computerisation of records with systems that meet with NHS approval; computer use should be integrated into consultations
- effective practice management
- appropriate availability of hospital services
- a practice library and other teaching aids including a video recorder to facilitate formative and summative assessments
- a volume of practice workload which ensures a balance for the GP registrar between the gaining of clinical experience and other opportunities for learning
- appropriate methods of responding to patient comments and complaints.

Prospective trainers should obtain a copy of their deanery's own criteria in addition to reading the JCPTGP's guidance.

Attracting a registrar

Because of the implications of the MADEL transfer, GP trainers are not now required to advertise for potential GP registrars nationally, or across Europe or the rest of the world! It is, however, important that the trainer attracts an appropriate GP registrar from the pool available following the central selection procedures. There continues to be a surplus of training practices over the number of registrars available. This means that the registrars will continue to have a choice of where to spend their training placement. It is important therefore that trainers consider how best to market their practice. Most deaneries are developing websites which will include details of all training practices, but why not consider designing your own? Trainers may also wish to consider the following:

▶ Develop your product: ensure you have an excellent, varied and attractive training practice and programme.
▶ Develop 'bonus offers' skills: are you a summative assessment assessor? MRCGP examiner? Do you have special skills that you teach? Acupuncture? Homeopathy? Clinical specialities?
▶ Consider the market's needs: can you reduce your on-call rota? If you are remote can you provide accommodation?
▶ Consider your resources and use past registrars (ask them to recommend). Be proactive (consider ringing potential applicants). Be visible and active where there are registrars (half-day release, joint trainer/registrar sessions, SHO programmes). Develop links with other practices for exchanges/shared posts.
▶ Flexibility: be prepared to take part-time applicants/job shares/varying length of posts.
▶ Develop your own market: have links with medical schools.

Summary comments

The detail of how to become a trainer can be overwhelming and the amount of paperwork generated by the deanery offices is enormous. A training practice will need a good system to keep up to date with the regulations and the paperwork. It is, however, well worth the effort in the end.

Appendix to Chapter 2

Minor surgery experience declaration

This is to certify that Dr .... has been a GP registrar in this practice from .... to .... He/She has attended an approved minor surgery theoretical course. He/She has received practical training and assessment in the following procedures:

(insert relevant procedures)

Dr .... (GP trainer)

Practice ....

Date ....

Child health surveillance experience declaration

This is to certify that Dr .... has been a GP registrar in this practice from ....
to .... and received at least six sessions of training in child health surveillance. He/She has attended an approved child health surveillance theoretical course.

Dr .... (GP trainer)

Practice ....

Date ....

Model contract

DR ....

AND

DR ....

AGREEMENT FOR TRAINING IN GENERAL PRACTICE

....

....

Note: The Implementation Group for the new UK GP Registrar Scheme is working on a new contract for GP Registrars and it is currently being discussed by the Department of Health and the BMA. It will supersede the BMA contract as presented here and will be available in early 2001. It can be accessed on the Internet via www.doh.gov.uk/medicaltrainingintheuk.

THIS AGREEMENT is made the ....
day of .... between ....
Medical Practitioner of .... Surgery
(hereafter called the 'Trainer') of the one part and
.... Medical Practitioner (hereafter
called the 'Registrar') of the other part.

WHEREAS:

(a) The parties are both practitioners fully registered with
the General Medical Council the Trainer being in General
Medical Practice at ....
....
(b) The Trainer having been appointed a Trainer by the
appropriate authorities and the Registrar being desirous of
the establishment of this contract upon the terms and
conditions hereinafter mentioned.

THESE BEING:

General

1 The Trainer undertakes to employ the Registrar and
   undertakes to instruct the Registrar in all aspects of
   General Practice and agrees to set aside regular periods
   for tuition (to total at least three hours per week on
   average) for a period of .... months unless
   the Agreement is terminated under the provisions of
   clause 2.

2 This Agreement can be terminated by the Registrar
   giving one calendar month's notice in writing to the
   Trainer or by the Trainer giving one calendar month's
   notice in writing to the Registrar and such notice may
   be given at any time.
   (a) The Trainer shall pay to the Registrar a salary and
   car allowance at the rates laid down from time to time
   in the Statement of Fees and Allowances payable to
   General Practitioners in England and Wales under the
   National Health Service Regulations. All payments will

be made in arrears at the end of each completed calendar month.

(b) The Registrar will be subject to the NHS Superannuation Regulations and the Trainer will deduct from the Registrar's salary and account to the proper authority for all contributions or payments for which the Registrar is liable under these regulations.

3 Both parties shall become and remain members of a recognised Medical Defence body at their own expense for the period of this Agreement.

4 All fees received by the Registrar by virtue of his/her position in the Practice shall be paid to the Trainer or as he may direct but any specific or pecuniary legacy or any gift of a specific chattel shall be the personal property of the Registrar.

5 The Registrar's hours of work in the Practice, the training programme and regular periods of tuition shall be agreed between the Registrar and the Trainer, making provision for appropriate day release and other commitments in accordance with the advice of the General Practice Advisory Committee and the Committee for Postgraduate Education in England. The Registrar's hours of work in the Practice both during and outside normal working hours shall not exceed the average hours of work in the Practice of members of the partnership or group.

6 (a) The Registrar shall be entitled to 30 working days' holiday during the period of 12 months and pro rata for shorter periods and general national holidays or days in lieu.

(b) The Registrar shall be entitled to 30 days approved study leave including attendance at day release courses on full pay and allowances during the 12-month period or pro rata for shorter periods. Additional study leave may be negotiated between the Registrar and Trainer subject to approval by the Regional Advisor in General Practice.

(c) If the Registrar is absent due to sickness the Trainer will pay over to him/her such sums as the trainer may receive from the Registrar's salary and board and lodging in accordance with the Statement of Fees and Allowances.

Duties and Responsibilities

7 (a) The Trainer undertakes to provide cover either by him/herself or by another Principal or vocationally-trained partner or assistant whenever the Registrar undertakes surgeries or on-call duties.

(b) The Trainer undertakes to provide the Registrar with such medical equipment and supplies (including drugs) as is agreed between them to be necessary for the proper execution of the Registrar's duties. The Registrar undertakes to take responsibility for the care and maintenance and if necessary replacement and return of such medical equipment and supplies at the end of the training period with the Trainer.

8 (a) The Registrar shall not, without the consent of the Trainer, undertake any duties or professional activities outside those of the Practice whether remunerated or not.

(b) The Registrar shall agree an educational programme with the Trainer and apply himself/herself diligently to this programme and to service commitments and other matters as directed by the Trainer in accordance with the advice of the Regional Director of Postgraduate GP Education.

(c) The Registrar shall preserve the confidentiality of the affairs of the Trainer, his/her partners, the patients and all matters connected with the Practice with the exception of the provision of certain information which may be requested by the Regional General Practice Subcommitee or Regional General Practice Director.

(d) The Registrar shall keep proper records of attendance and visits by and to any patients and all other such records as are reasonably required by the Trainer.

(e) The Registrar will be required to live in lodgings agreed as suitable by the Trainer while on-call.

(f) The Registrar will provide, maintain and pay all the running costs of suitable transport to enable him/her efficiently to carry out his/her responsibilities under this Agreement.

Miscellaneous

9 For a period of three years, or such period as accepted by both parties or deemed appropriate by an agreed third party in the event of a failure to reach agreement, following the completion of the training programme the Registrar unless practising in the Trainer's Practice will not:

(a) accept on his/her own list any patient who during the training programme was on the NHS lists of the Trainer or one of his partners

(b) attend or treat, unless in emergency, in the capacity of a General Medical Practitioner any such patient as is mentioned in (a) above

(c) recommend any such patient to seek inclusion on the NHS lists of any Medical Practitioner other than the Trainer or one of his/her partners. This clause shall be effective only in relation to such patients who during the period of the training programme resided within a radius of five miles from the building known as the .... surgery and each of the sub-clauses (a), (b) and (c) shall be separately enforceable as if independent covenants.

10 Any dispute between the parties or those in any way representing them concerning this Agreement or the

employment of the Registrar or anything arising from this Agreement shall be referred to a sole arbitrator under the Arbitration Act 1950 nominated by the Secretary of the British Medical Association providing always that any dispute relating to education and training shall be referred to the Regional Director of Postgraduate General Practice Education for referral to the General Practice Subcommittee of the Regional Postgraduate Education Committee whose decision shall be final and binding on all the parties concerned.

11 The terms of this contract will be subject to the Terms of Service for doctors as set out from time to time in the National Health Service (General Medical and Pharmaceutical Services) Regulations.

AS WITNESS the hands of the parties hereto the day and year before written.

SIGNED by the said ....

In the presence of ....

SIGNED by the said ....

In the presence of ....

Form VTR2

NATIONAL HEALTH SERVICE **VTR/2 (Jan 98)**
Vocational Training for General Practice

STATEMENT OF SATISFACTORY COMPLETION
OF A PERIOD OF TRAINING IN AN
EDUCATIONALLY APPROVED POST
(A separate form must be completed
for each post held)

Dr (full name) _____

General Medical Council
  Full Registration No. _____

National GP Registrar No. _____

Address _____

has, for the purposes of the National Health Service
(Vocational Training for General Medical Practice) and
European Requirements (Amendment) Regulations, 1997,
satisfactorily completed the period of training detailed
below:

...... months, From ...... day ...... month ...... year, To
...... day ...... month ...... year as a registered practitioner
in the following approved training post:

Hospital _____ Post No. _____
Grade _____ Specialty _____
Address of hospital _____

Please delete as appropriate:
* the training was whole-time
* the training was part-time and the ratio of part-time to
  whole-time was _____

Name _____ HOSPITAL STAMP

(consultant or other medical specialist
of similar status who has supervised the
practitioner's training)

Signed _____

Post/Rank _____

Date _____

ENDORSEMENT BY DIRECTOR OF
POSTGRADUATE GENERAL PRACTICE
EDUCATION OR NOMINATED DEPUTY

Dr _____, *Regional Director,*

_____ *Region*

Directors of Postgraduate General Practice Education:

After signature, this form should be returned to the doctor named above for safekeeping.

Doctors training for general practice:

You will need to send this form to the JCPTGP, 14 Princes Gate, Hyde Park, London SW7 1PU (Tel 020 7581 3232) with your VTR/1 and other VTR/2 forms, and a copy of your GMC registration certificate. Please enclose a letter quoting your full name and address for correspondence.

VTR/2 (Jan 98)

Note 1 – Satisfactory completion is defined in Regulation 9(1). It means, in relation to a period of training in any employment, the completion of that period of training in such a manner as to have acquired the medical experience which may reasonably be expected to be acquired from training of that duration in that employment.

Note 2 – Part-time training is defined in Regulation 7 as follows:

(a) in computing any period of training which began on or before 31 December 1994 there shall be disregarded any period of part-time employment during which the duties of the person employed occupied less than half of the time usually occupied by the duties of persons employed whole-time in similar employment; and

(b) in computing any period of training which began after 31 December 1994 there shall be disregarded any period of part-time employment during which the duties of the person employed, taken week by week, occupied less than 60% of the time usually occupied by the duties of persons employed whole-time in similar employment;

and in relation to any period of training which began after 31 December 1994 employment which is not whole-time shall not be regarded as equivalent to whole-time employment unless it includes at least two periods of whole-time employment each lasting not less than one week, one such period falling within paragraph (3) [training as a GP registrar] and one within paragraph (4) [training in hospital posts].

Note 3 – Approval of training posts. The approval of hospital posts is defined in regulation 8(2):

The Joint Committee may approve a post for the purposes of paragraph (1) if:

(a) it is approved by the Specialist Training Authority of the Medical Royal Colleges pursuant to Article 7 of the European Specialist Medical Qualifications Order 1995(b); or

(b) it is not so approved and the post is one for which there is no relevant Royal College or Faculty.

This form is produced by the JCPTGP. January 1998

Form VTR1

Vocational Training for General Practice

STATEMENT OF SATISFACTORY COMPLETION OF A PERIOD OF TRAINING AS A GP REGISTRAR

(A separate form must be completed
for each post held)

Dr (full name) _____

General Medical Council
    Full Registration No. _____

National GP Training No. _____

Address _____

has, for the purposes of the National Health Service (Vocational Training for General Medical Practice) and European Requirements (Amendment) Regulations, 1997, satisfactorily completed the period of training detailed below:

...... months, From ...... day ...... month ...... year, To ...... day ...... month ...... year as a GP Registrar under my instruction and supervision.

Please delete as appropriate:
* the training was whole-time
* the training was part-time and the ratio of part-time to whole-time was _____

Signed _____ Date _____

(an approved General Practice trainer)

TRAINER'S NAME
AND PRACTICE
ADDRESS
_____
_____
_____
_____
_____
_____

ENDORSEMENT OF
THE TRAINER'S
SIGNATURE BY
DIRECTOR OF
POSTGRADUATE
GENERAL PRACTICE
EDUCATION OR
NOMINATED DEPUTY

_____

Dr _____ ,
    Regional Director
DATE _____

TO BE COMPLETED BY THE DIRECTOR OF
POSTGRADUATE GENERAL PRACTICE
EDUCATION ON COMPLETION OF THE FINAL
PERIOD IN GENERAL PRACTICE

I certify that she/he has passed all elements of summative
assessment as laid down by the Joint Committee on
Postgraduate Training for General Practice:

Signed _____ Date _____

Dr _____ , *Regional Director,*

_____ *Region*

Directors of Postgraduate General Practice Education:

After signature, this form should be returned to the
trainee named above for safekeeping.

GP Registrars:

You will need to send this form to the JCPTGP,
14 Princes Gate, Hyde Park, London SW7 1PU

(Tel 020 7581 3232) with any other VTR/1 forms, your VTR/2 forms and a copy of your GMC registration certificate. Please enclose a letter quoting your full name and address for correspondence.

VTR/1 (Jan 98)

Note 1 – Satisfactory completion is defined in Regulation 9(1). It means, in relation to a period of training in any employment, the completion of that period of training in such a manner as to have acquired the medical experience which may reasonably be expected to be acquired from training of that duration in that employment.

Note 2 – Part-time training is defined in Regulation 7 as follows:

(a) in computing any period of training which began on or before 31 December 1994 there shall be disregarded any period of part-time employment during which the duties of the person employed occupied less than half of the time usually occupied by the duties of persons employed whole-time in similar employment; and

(b) in computing any period of training which began after 31 December 1994 there shall be disregarded any period of part-time employment during which the duties of the person employed, taken week by week, occupied less than 60% of the time usually occupied by the duties of persons employed whole-time in similar employment;

and in relation to any period of training which began after 31 December 1994 employment which is not whole-time shall not be regarded as equivalent to whole-time employment unless it includes at least two periods of whole-time employment each lasting not less than one week, one such period falling within paragraph (3) [training as a GP registrar] and one within paragraph (4) [training in hospital posts].

Note 3 – Attestation to completion of summative assessment. Some trainees split the period of training as a GP registrar into one or more terms. The section of the form attesting to the passing of summative assessment need only be completed at the stage when the GP registrar has passed all elements of summative assessment.

Note 4 – Approval of trainers. The approval of trainers is defined in regulation 7:

(1) A practitioner [is approved if]:
  (a) his name is included in a medical list; and
  (b) he is for the time being approved by the Joint Committee ...
(2) An approval under paragraph (1) may be withdrawn by the Joint Committee at any time before it expires.
(3) The Joint Committee must, before approving a practitioner ... be satisfied that the characteristics and qualities of the practitioner and his practice are such that he is suitable to provide the experience referred to in regulation 6(3).

This form is produced by the JCPTGP. January 1998

CHAPTER 3

Learning needs assessment: how do trainers assess the learning needs of registrars?

'Aller Anfang ist schwer' – all beginnings are hard

German proverb

Introduction

What is our role as trainers in postgraduate primary care education? Some light can be shed on this complex question by looking at the various terms used to describe the post. In the UK, we are trainers – this implies we should be training! Training has connotations of directing, leading and informing. In Australia, supervisors and educators take on the role together. This seems to suggest a monitoring and educational element. In Canada, the term used is preceptor. This implies a person who has gone on before and has experience – perhaps as a role model. The educational world would like to call us all facilitators – someone to make things easier for the trainee, registrar, resident or learner (we won't go into these!). In fact, our role encompasses all of these elements

– the semantics reveal a breadth and flexibility of role that 'trainers' need to aspire to achieve. This, however, is a practical manual and despite the potential beauty of semantics most of these terms are used interchangeably.

Perhaps one further comment on these semantics does bear repeating. There are a number of potential traps that 'teachers' can fall into. These can best be summarised in four statement fallacies:

- ► teachers know everything
- ► teachers can do everything well
- ► all you need to do to learn is copy the teacher (the God syndrome)
- ► teachers show you how to do it, i.e. 'look how brilliant I am' (fostering dependence).

Perhaps facilitators, educators, trainers or supervisors don't do any of these things!

This chapter covers the methods trainers use to assess the learning needs of registrars. The section aims to provide a description of the tools trainers are using in the assessment of educational needs, a brief description of where they seem to be useful and, finally, how to get your hands on them if you want to have a go.

A wide range of methods were employed to assess the educational needs of registrars. These methods attempt to balance the conflicting needs of a registrar/learner-centred programme with those of a professionally determined curriculum of ill-defined nature. They cover a range of knowledge, skills and attitudinal assessments. Various approaches to defining the curriculum are described in Chapter 5.

Most trainers facilitated a process of self-assessment by the learner in accordance with the principles of adult learning. Many trainers felt the need to offer structural guidance in the form of various confidence rating scales, checklists, tests of knowledge and other questionnaires. Many of these are described in the following sections.

Needs assessment of knowledge

Wolverhampton Grid	Regional documentation	MCQs
Confidence rating scales	Manchester rating scales	Other techniques

Learner-based self-rating confidence lists relating to the medical curriculum

- ► Wolverhampton Grid (revised 1999)
  – an in-depth look at skills and knowledge in a lengthy scale (*see* Appendix A).

- ► Documentation provided by the deaneries
  – most deaneries produce formative assessment packages with rating scales that the learner can self-score.

- ► Confidence rating scales
  – initial educational planning list (*see* Appendix A). A short scoring list covering both basic and more advanced areas
  – the Combined Confidence Rating Scale (*see* Appendix A). This is the result of combining a number of practice-designed rating scales. The result is a practical list, shorter than the Wolverhampton Grid, that still covers most areas.

Comments: these lists attempt to assess needs and cover a recognised 'core' of areas. They will often help the development of the initial educational plan for the new registrar. They can appear daunting to some registrars, generally do not prioritise learning needs and need careful introduction. The Wolverhampton Grid was mentioned most frequently but is a rather lengthy list with some questionable inclusions. It is helpful to ask a number of experienced GPs (partners, colleagues) to complete these forms, and to keep copies of past registrars' forms, to provide benchmarks of 'normal' confidence levels. This can demonstrate to the registrar that no one expects them to be completely confident in all areas.

Trainer/facilitator-based rating methods

► Manchester rating scales
  – RCGP occasional paper 40 available from RCGP.

► Documentation from the deanery
  – as mentioned above this is primarily designed in most deaneries for the trainer's use.

Comments: the Manchester rating scales are not popular with trainers – only 7% mentioned them. Used as a whole they are a cumbersome tool. Selective use can be a different process and is described in Chapter 6.

MCQ-based assessment

► Phased evaluation programme (PEP)
  – available from the RCGP (can be downloaded directly via the internet) or ring 020 7581 3232.

Comment: this is a very useful collection of MCQ/MEQ-type questions available for computer use. The basic programme involves a bank of validated questions similar to the MRCGP MCQ examination. It provides a printed result of the learner's performance. This is broken down into scores in particular areas (i.e. therapeutics, ENT, etc.) and the learner's scores compared with 200 other registrar scores. It can be used to assess the need for work on the knowledge base and also to boost confidence for examinations (summative assessment particularly). Two generalised versions are in existence so the process can be repeated to demonstrate improvement. Additional programmes are now available on more specific areas (health and safety, practice management, etc.).

▶ Other MCQ resources

Comment: trainers mentioned a number of sources for these – the examination handbooks (*see* book list Chapter 12), cuttings from various publications (*Pulse*, *GP*, *Medicine International*, etc.) and past examinations. One technique was to batch these in subject areas and use them in tutorials as a teaching and assessment tool.

▶ Other IT resources
  – MCQ master (*see* Appendix A).

Comment: it seems likely that the current generation of trainers are not as aware as they might be (or as their registrars are!) of the educational opportunities that are developing in this area. MCQ master is a computer program that enables you to enter your own questions (and answers!) with accompanying comments. It is designed for self-use but does print out score results. It has obvious educational value as well as a needs assessment potential. It does, however, require a bank of questions and quite a lot of initial work to enter these.

Other techniques

▶ MEQ questions
▶ case analysis
▶ video
▶ role play
▶ sitting in
▶ script analysis
▶ referral analysis
▶ critical event analysis
▶ joint visits
▶ note review.

Comments: all of these techniques were mentioned and have the potential to assess knowledge. They also have the potential to leave areas unsampled if used alone.

They involve more realistic settings (i.e. have process validity) and often feel more relevant to both registrar and trainer. These methods are unlikely to result in objective measurements of knowledge, but much of general practice seems to have a 'gut-weighted' element and many trainers feel this is probably valid.

Assessment of skill

Skills list I to III	Self-perception inventory	Personality tests
Thinking styles	Learning styles	Interpersonal skill assessment tools
Assertion skills	Motivation tools	

Trainers found the needs assessment for this area more difficult and much of the assessment was based on direct observation or the reports of others. The following resources were mentioned.

Skills checklists

A number of these are printed in Appendix A. They are a curricular approach to skills assessment and allow an overview of past learning and future needs. Appendix A includes lists relating to clinical and management/administrative skills.

Self-awareness needs assessment methods

A number of techniques were mentioned in this area. Most of these are commercially available questionnaire-based tools and are mentioned below with brief comments.

Self-awareness needs

- Self-perception inventory (Belbin 1981)
- Learning style questionnaire (Honey and Mumford 1992)
- Personality styles (Firo B, Personality styles, Crown Crisp, Myers–Briggs)
- Thinking styles
- Interpersonal styles (Honey and Mumford 1992)
- Influencing styles (Honey and Mumford 1992)
- Win–win questionnaire (Honey and Mumford 1992)
- Counselling styles (Honey and Mumford 1992)
- Miller–Smith lifestyle assessment
- Assertion rights questionnaire
- Motivation rank order scale.

Comment: brief notes based on trainers' comments for each of these resources follows below. Information on how to acquire these questionnaires is included in Appendix A.

Self-perception inventory: developed by Belbin (1981), this questionnaire allocates a score reflecting your team role strengths. The categories are:

- chairperson – director
- company worker – practical and efficient
- completer/finisher – task-orientated driving force
- monitor/evaluator – analytical and checking
- resource investigator – looks externally for resources
- teamworker – supportive
- shaper – looks at objectives and outcome
- plant – looks for novel solutions.

A lot of trainers have found this useful. At the assessment level it gives the trainer an insight into the registrar's normal team behaviour and raises awareness of team functions.

Learning style questionnaire: this is a questionnaire developed by Honey and Mumford. Peter Honey is a psychologist who has produced a prolific number of self-awareness questionnaires of varying use in the training period. Most trainers feel that this one has the greatest value. It gives you a learning style in one of the following four categories:

▶ Reflectors – good at thinking over the implications but slow to act.
▶ Theorists – good at analysing/explaining, but tendency to be unrealistic.
▶ Pragmatists – eager for the practical approach, but can miss other implications.
▶ Activists – eager to get on with the 'doing' but at the expense of thinking.

The manual includes detailed descriptions of learning styles and provides useful advice on how to maximise the value of a particular style and how to improve weaker styles. It is possible to structure the training programme to reflect the registrar's style and many trainers feel this has been successful, i.e. more 'hands on' with the activist, more 'models' for the theorist, etc.

Personality styles: trainers need to be cautious using these tools – they can facilitate learning and the development of self-awareness but they can also penetrate the defences of vulnerable individuals and cause harm. They seem to be used at two levels: first, as a 'fun' tool to explore the issues around personality and the caring role, and second, to look at a potential problem. If they are used for this second purpose the trainer should consider the following questions:

▶ Do I have the registrar's permission/consent to do this?
▶ Have I considered the potential for harm?
▶ Have I been explicit with the registrar about the purpose of this?
▶ Do both the registrar and I share an agreed agenda?
▶ How am I going to 'safety net' the process?

Having considered all this, four types of personality-style indicators were mentioned by trainers:

▶ The Firo B personality test is a scale that measures three parameters of your **F**undamental **I**nterpersonal **R**elationship **O**rientation in a **B**ehavioural context. It looks at inclusion, control and affection areas. If a registrar appears to have a problem in these areas, the tool can help analyse this situation. It can highlight difficulties with the need to relax control, handle unexpressed emotion or to look at detached behaviour.

▶ The Crown Crisp experiential index is a simple personality index with a more clinically orientated basis. It is an indicator of personality traits and can be fun to complete. It gives a personality trait score in the following areas:
  – anxious
  – depressive
  – phobic
  – hysterical
  – obsessional
  – somatic.
If the trainer feels it would be helpful to explore these personality traits then this tool offers a method of achieving this.

▶ The Personality style inventory places you on a grid between these four extremes:
  – enthusiast: enjoys feelings and doing
  – imaginative: enjoys feelings and intuiting
  – practical: enjoys doing and thinking
  – logical: enjoys thinking and intuiting.
Guidance is then offered on the basis of your placement on the grid.

▶ The Myers–Briggs type indicator classifies interaction styles into four bipolar scales:
  – what you pay attention to: sensing–intuition scale
  – how you are energised: introversion–
                               extroversion scale

– how you live and work: perceiving–judging scale
– how you make decisions: thinking–feeling scale.
This can help in the assessment of learning style (published by Consulting Psychologists Press Inc., 3803 East Bayshore Road, Palo Alto, California 94303, USA). A useful summary of key elements is included in the Appendix to Chapter 1.

These tools are probably best used as a light-hearted and less threatening way of looking at how our personalities affect behaviour. This has particular implications for learning, consulting and team role areas.

Thinking styles I: this is a simple model dividing learners into three groups:

▶ dreamers
▶ realists
▶ critics/evaluators.

This can have implications for the methodology used in training.

Thinking styles II: Neame (1984) describes two main thinking styles: the serialist and the holist. The serialist tends to learn by analysing the problem and organising thought in a sequential manner. Information gathering and problem solving is encouraged by facilitating this process, i.e. chopping material into blocks that can be linked and led towards the goal. This thought process starts at the bottom and works upwards. It is comprehensive but can also be laborious and slow. Holistic thinkers look at the whole picture and try to deduce solutions based on the sum of the available parts without dissecting them. This tends to be a quicker process but is in danger of making assumptions and bending observations to 'fit the picture'. Holistic thinkers can be helped by highlighting features of the problem and encouraging a 'safety netting' process where they are encouraged to look for evidence that has either been ignored or contradicts their position.

Interpersonal styles: places the individual on an autocratic/democratic negotiation line. It is primarily aimed at industrial management trainees and seems a little naive, but could be useful as an assessment of interpersonal attitudes. It may help the registrar who has difficulty negotiating appropriate management options with patients.

Influencing styles: introduces the idea of directive, collaborative and consultative styles. This seems to have value in assessing a registrar's style and attitude to staff management. It may also have a role in assessing negotiation skills within the consultation. In this sense it will help in needs assessments/problem definition in these areas.

Win–win questionnaire: this questionnaire looks at the attitudes and behaviour necessary to achieve win–win situations. It would probably have most use where a registrar seemed to be having a problem in negotiation, particularly where he/she or the other party were consistently 'losers'. In this situation it would help clarify the problem and define areas of need.

Counselling style: this is a simplistic analysis of counselling looking specifically at the skills of non-directive counselling. It seems to offer little but may help in the needs assessment of a registrar who was struggling with the counselling role at an early stage in training.

Miller–Smith lifestyle assessment: this is a questionnaire designed to look at the stress level inherent in one's current lifestyle. It allows an assessment of the learner's capacity to take on new challenges involving further stress. It can also help analyse current stressors and suggest stress reduction solutions.

Assertion rights questionnaire: this can produce a needs assessment of assertiveness skills and attitudes. It involves the 'OK' principles, i.e. 'you're OK, I'm OK' or 'you're OK, I'm not OK', and all the other permutations. It is discussed further in Chapter 7.

Motivation rank order scale: this is a list of motivating values the individual places in a rank order that reflects his or her feelings. It can be an eye-opening experience that helps understand motivation and develop learning needs in this area. The details are in the appendix to this chapter.

Trainer/facilitator-based rating methods

▶ Summary sheet (*see* Appendix A).

Comment: needs assessment was often based on discussion with the registrar in the light of his or her past experience. This is an essential element but has the capacity to be incomplete and imprecise. The summary sheet seems to offer a structure that seeks to remedy this. Consultation needs assessment was very closely linked to the consultation skills teaching process (as discussed in the introduction to this chapter). This area is covered in Chapter 4.

Needs assessment of attitudes

Attribute lists	Manchester rating scales	Attitudinal lists
Ethical scenarios		

The definition and assessment of attitudes in registrars is a difficult area. Often trainers will be aware of a problem but find it difficult to define, with justification, exactly where the problem lies. The desirable attributes of a GP were defined by Battles *et al.* (1990) and are shown in Table 3.1. This list can be used as a guide to try and identify where problems lie.

Most trainers seem to assess registrars' attitudinal needs by observation and discussion of video-taped consultations, role playing particular scenarios, problem patient discussion and ethical dilemma discussions. There was little structural component evident in most of these

Table 3.1: The attributes of the ideal primary care physician (from Battles *et al.* 1990)

Communication skills	Relationships with patients	Personal attributes	Professional attitudes
1 Can communicate	1 Demonstrates care and concern	1 Empathic and understanding	1 Competent
2 Is a good listener			2 Compassionate
3 Has professional respect for individual worth regardless of social status, moral values, economic status or lifestyle	2 Interested in patients	2 Has common sense	3 Professional
	3 Accepts different patients	3 Honesty	4 Respectful
	4 Exhibits patience	4 Has integrity	5 Confident
	5 Has rapport with patients	5 Courteous	6 Flexible
	6 Has empathy for families	6 Sensitive	7 Comprehensive
	7 Comforting	7 Possesses wisdom	8 Persistent
	8 Uses self-restraint	8 Optimistic	9 Compulsive
	9 Supportive	9 Humble	10 Willing and able to work in a team
	10 Can formulate goals and ways to meet them	10 Accepts own mortality	11 Interested in human nature, enjoying the beauty in each person
		11 Firm	12 Curious and keeps up to date
		12 Shows love	
		13 Tolerant	

activities. The following resources were used in some practices:

▶ registrar attitudinal rating scale (*see* Appendix A)
▶ sections of the Manchester rating scales (particularly 19–23)
▶ ethical scenarios (*see* Appendix A).

Other methods for assessing needs

Diaries	PUNS/DENS	Note review
Personal construct analysis	Wish list	Others

A variety of other methods were mentioned and are described briefly:

▶ Diary use – many trainers suggest that the registrar keeps an educational diary.

Comment: the technique suggested for using the diary determines its usefulness to the registrar. The following advice can help:

– have the diary open on the desk for every surgery
– write two comments per surgery
– record difficult patients
– write down any questions that occur to you
– bring the diary to every tutorial.

An introduction to the idea of reflective learning (*see* Chapter 5) can be helpful for the registrar. Limiting the diary to an 'emotional' diary (*see* Chapter 10) for recording the feeling that certain patients produce can highlight attitudinal problems. Certainly to be useful the trainer must regularly review its contents for most registrars.

▶ PUNS and DENS – Patient Unmet Needs and Doctor's Educational Needs.

Comment: this acronym was developed at Taunton by Richard Eve and is really a simple system to aid reflective experiential learning. After each consultation the registrar is encouraged to record any patient needs they felt they had not managed well. The trainer looks at these and helps the registrar convert them into educational needs.

▶ 20-note review.

Comment: many trainers review notes for a variety of reasons. The form in the appendix to this chapter was suggested as a method of structuring this process. Certainly this approach can generate an agenda for learning needs.

▶ Personal construct analysis.

Comment: this is a technique for encouraging the registrar to declare his or her own perceived strengths and weaknesses in any particular area. It usually involves asking him or her to list perhaps the 10 most easy and 10 most difficult scenarios for them in a given area, i.e. produced for a specific condition (asthma) or situation (angry patients).

It seems to add another perspective if the trainer produces his or her own lists too. Often the similarities are reassuring for registrars and the differences provoke some interesting discussion. Further details are provided in Chapter 10.

▶ Registrar wish list (*see* Appendix A).

Comment: this is simply a written record of what the registrar would like to achieve. It can be useful to revisit this list from time to time. It does serve to emphasise the learner-centred philosophy and encourage the registrar's contribution at an early stage.

Trainers also mentioned a number of other stimuli to the development of learning needs:

▶ Feedback from patients, staff and partners (*see* Appendix A).

Comment: it was not clear how reliable trainers felt these sources were or how the comments were recorded (if at all). Some trainers kept their own diary for making brief notes. This would seem a practical way to monitor whether there were any trends in comments from people that might suggest a learning need.

▶ Analysis of prescriptions.

Comment: this can be achieved directly in dispensing practices or by carboning prescriptions, the use of computer printouts or PACT data. PACT data for registrars can be provided separately by marking their scripts with a red T. However, the data are slow to arrive and not one trainer made a positive comment on this approach.

Summary comments

Many trainers specifically commented on the need to produce the right atmosphere in the practice for the process of needs assessment to work effectively. This raises two questions: first, what is the *right* atmosphere?, and second, how do you produce it?

Characteristics of the *right* atmosphere seem to include:

▶ a non-threatening environment
▶ a good teacher–learner relationship
▶ a learner-centred approach
▶ the potential for excitement or fun
▶ the opportunity to apply new learning
▶ the availability of a good standard for learners to assess themselves against
▶ opportunities exist for the learner to be aware of their role in facilitating the learning in others
▶ learners are aware of their progress towards their own learning goals.

The 'Holy Grail' concept is an interesting enhancement to the learning atmosphere. Throughout history humans have been highly motivated by 'visions' of unseen and exciting possibilities. In down-to-earth terms, educators can encourage this by introducing novelty and experiment in their programmes and by deliberately encouraging dreaming and ambition in the process.

More insights to help trainers produce the *right* atmosphere come from the concepts of role modelling, effective supervision and constructive feedback. The characteristics of these are described in McEvoy's *Educating the Future GP* (1998) and summarised in Table 3.2.

This section has aimed to provide practical methods and food for thought in the needs assessment of registrars. It is an area that offers a huge variety of methods that should make the process stimulating.

Table 3.2: Characteristics of role modelling, effective supervision and constructive feedback

Characteristics of role modelling	Characteristics of effective supervision	Characteristics of constructive feedback

► teacher exhibits enthusiasm
► self-confident in his/her abilities
► demonstrates awareness of his/her strengths/weaknesses
► shares his/her struggles and successes as a learning process
► effect on patient care of learning process acknowledged
► uses modelling role to:
  – demonstrate skills
  – influence attitudes
► is open to criticism as a learning opportunity
► exhibits a planned approach to teaching
► is open in setting objectives
	► teacher selects appropriate learning experiences
	► highlights learning objectives
	► accessibility discussed and defined
	► supervision level discussed and defined
		► highlights effective/ineffective behaviours
		► provides descriptive and specific feedback
		► feedback involves sharing of information
		► feedback is not overwhelming
		► teacher is aware of the effects of feedback on the learner
		► feedback avoids collusion, i.e. is honest

CHAPTER 4

Teaching consultation skills: how do trainers teach consultation skills?

Communication is the most important tool the physician can possess. Learn to respect it and use it wisely

Meador

Introduction

Most trainers feel that the development of a registrar's interest in consultation skills is the crux of the GP training year. To raise the registrar's awareness of the communication dynamics at work in the consultation and to see them developing these skills is for most of us a tremendously rewarding experience. But how do trainers do this? Read on!

This chapter describes the techniques trainers use to teach consultation skills. These methods can be grouped into those involving patients or patient scenarios (video, role play or joint consultations) and those using other resources.

The last element of this chapter looks at the assessment of consulting skills.

Patient contact-related methods

Use of video

Not surprisingly, video was the most common tool used, but how is it used? A number of strategies were mentioned.

Consultation mapping (*see* Appendix to this chapter)

Comment: This is a process of categorising what is happening in the consultation. Until recently it was required for a number of consultations submitted for the MRCGP examination. It can lead to the interpretation that the consultation should progress through this sequence of events to produce a satisfactory outcome. Most trainers feel that this is a questionable assumption. (Notice the use of the word assume: it makes an ASS out of U and ME!) However, it can be an interesting tool to use if the registrar seems to be struggling with the structure of the consultation and it does cover all the major elements one would hope to see.

Consultation modelling

Comment: Some trainers feel consultation models are about as much use in teaching consultation skills as Airfix models are if you want to fly! However, many would not share that view. A good description of the models is available from many sources and the book section contains the relevant references. The different models have different perspectives that lend themselves to teaching consultation skills in different areas of need. The following is a brief description of each:

▸ **The RCGP model** simply asks the doctor to look beyond the organic and include the psychosocial elements of presentations and ill health.

Physical, psychological and social – encourages the doctor to extend his or her thinking into these dimensions with each presentation.

▸ **Stott and Davis's 1979 model** is very task-orientated. Many trainers feel a fifth task (are there any administrative elements to this consultation?) should be added to the four original ones. This can be a useful model to expand the registrar's outlook, particularly into the realms of prevention. It has no overtly psychodynamic elements and many trainers felt this was a major drawback.

- Management of presenting problems
- Modification of help-seeking behaviour
- Management of continuing problems
- Opportunistic health promotion (administrative element).

▸ **Byrne and Long's 1976 model** is a mechanistic model that was derived from the analysis of many consultations. Their book is fairly short and has some interesting comments on dysfunctional consultations and attempts to change doctor behaviour (*see* Chapter 11). Most trainers felt the model had limited application in this area.

- Phase 1 – The doctor establishes a relationship with the patient.
- Phase 2 – The doctor attempts to discover the reason for the consultation.
- Phase 3 – The doctor conducts a verbal and/or physical examination.
- Phase 4 – The doctor, or the doctor and patient, or the patient consider the problem.
- Phase 5 – The doctor, and occasionally the patient, discuss management.
- Phase 6 – The consultation is terminated.

▶ **Pendleton *et al.*'s 1984 model** combines a structural element with a psychodynamic element and is the basis of many of the consultation maps around. *The Consultation: an approach to learning and teaching* is considered essential reading by many trainers and is undoubtedly useful in teaching consultation skills. Many trainers particularly mentioned Pendleton's rules described in the book as a method of giving feedback in the video-based tutorial. These will be described later in this section.

- Define the reason
  for attendance: – nature and history of problems
                – their aetiology
                – the patient's ideas/concerns/
                    expectations
                – the effects of the problem.
- Consider other
  problems: – continuing problems
           – at-risk factors.
- Choose an appropriate action for each problem.
- Achieve an understanding with the patient.
- Involve the patient in the management plan with some responsibility for it.
- Use time and resources appropriately.
- Establish/maintain the appropriate relationship.

▶ **Helman's 1984 model** is an anthropological model and helps registrars gain an insight into the patient's agenda. It is useful if the registrar seems to have a very doctor-centred approach.

- What has happened?
- Why has it happened? Why to me? Why now?
- What would happen if I did nothing?
- What should I do about it?
- What can you (the doctor) do about it?
- How can I stop it happening again?

▶ **Heron's 1986 six-category intervention analysis** is a model describing the range of interventions available to the doctor. It is useful when a registrar is having problems in the management of patients – particularly the 'difficult' patient.

- Prescriptive – advising/telling
- Informative – instructing/interpreting
- Confronting – challenging/feeding back
- Cathartic – releasing emotions
- Catalytic – encouraging exploration
- Supportive – comforting/affirming.

▶ **Berne's 1977 transactional analysis** is a model of human behaviour (child, adult, parent) and allows an interpretation of some situations that many registrars do find difficult.

- Ego-states – parent/child/adult.

▶ **Murtagh's 1998 model** is again a mechanistic model that has a pragmatic feel to it. It might prove useful to the anxious registrar in that it offers more concrete advice on the uncertainties of diagnosis. Many would feel this was not the ideal solution for dealing with this problem.

- What is the probability diagnosis?
- What serious diagnosis should not be missed?
- What conditions are often missed? (provides a list of conditions)
- Is this a 'masquerade'? (provides a list of conditions)
- Is the patient trying to tell me something I've missed?

▶ **The Cambridge–Calgary model** adopts an evidence-based approach to consultation skills teaching that will be described later in this chapter. It has a practical flavour that appeals to many trainers.

- Initiating the consultation
- Gathering information
- Building the relationship/facilitating the patient's involvement

- Explanation and planning
- Closing the consultation.

▶ **Neighbour's 1987 model** is widely used by trainers although it is not clear how practical the exercises suggested in the book are in reality. Its attraction seems to lie in the five key words of the model. Summarising, handing over, safety netting and housekeeping seem to have been particularly useful concepts. This will be looked at again later in this chapter.

1 – Connecting
2 – Summarising
3 – Handing over
4 – Safety netting
5 – Housekeeping.

In his book *The Inner Consultation*, Neighbour also introduces the idea of acceptance sets and calibration sets and some trainers found this useful. Patients often have particular patterns of body language in response to particular situations. If the doctor can identify the set for agreement (the acceptance set) or other situations (sadness, confusion, frustration, etc.) he or she can become calibrated to the patient and increase the chance of better communication. Certainly trainers can use the video to illustrate this phenomenon and raise registrar awareness.

▶ **Neurolinguistic programming** has developed a significant following in the USA. This is quite a complicated system based on models of how the brain handles information. If the communicator can identify the predominant system in the person they are communicating with, then it suggests ways of improving communication with them. Some trainers have found a number of the concepts useful:

– Dominant perceptual system theory states that people view the world from a kinaesthetic (feeling), visual (seeing) or auditory (hearing) point of view. They use and respond to words in their relevant system more readily. They also express their preference in other behaviours, i.e. the visual person will *see* something is wrong and might respond better to a pictorial explanation than a verbal one. If the doctor can use the patient's system he or she will feel better understood and treated. A particular exercise the trainer can use here is to ask registrars to repeat the advice they gave to the patient but particularly using the patient's own words and trying to use their particular system in some form. This concept is illustrated further in the Appendix to Chapter 2.

– Eye movement indicators are another concept that can be useful. People's eye movements seem to provide insight into thought processes. This is described in detail in *The Inner Consultation* by Neighbour (1987). Few people have been able to describe using this on a large scale but it is practical to learn the one or two common movements (i.e. those indicating a feeling or visual memory).

▶ **McWhinney's 1972 disease–illness model** draws a parallel between the traditional medical model of illness and a patient-centred perspective. This sort of process may help the registrar with a lot of hospital-based experience as it drafts a patient-centred perspective on to the skeleton of a well-established mode of thinking (*see* Figure 4.1).

McWhinney, a co-author of the model above (with Levenstein 1986), described a dual concept to help understand why a patient presents at a particular time. Patients reach either their 'limit of symptom tolerance' or their 'limit of anxiety'. If the doctor can understand which trigger is at work the consultation is more likely to be successful. This insight can help focus registrars on the patient agenda.

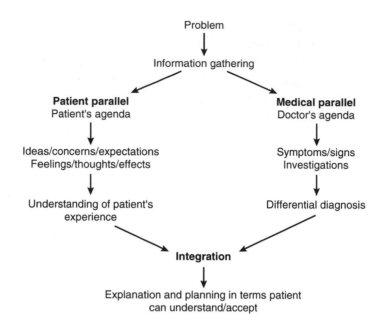

Figure 4.1: McWhinney's disease–illness model.

Constructive feedback methods

Pendleton's rules

Pendleton's rules remain a very useful and commonly employed tool. Some would argue that they are a little contrived and that registrars ignore the positive comments: 'everything before the but is crap' as someone more crudely put it. However, they are designed to be protective of the learner in a vulnerable situation and it is still the case that many registrars feel threatened by the video. In summary, the trainer runs through the following scheme after the video consultation:

▶ What do you think you did well?
▶ What do I think you did well?
▶ What do you think you could have done differently? (and how)

> ▸ What do I think you could have done differently? (and how)
> ▸ How do you feel about this?
> ▸ Finish on a positive reinforcement of good consultation behaviour.

SETGO method

The SETGO method is described in *Teaching and Learning Communication Skills in Medicine* by Silverman *et al.* (1998) (*see* Chapter 11). We all tend to be our own worst critics and this method enables the registrar to identify their own learning goals in a non-threatening way. Its major advantage lies in going straight to the points raised by the learner. Briefly the registrar and trainer look at the video and make observational notes where they think appropriate, but generally on a minute-to-minute basis. After the consultation the trainer facilitates the following process:

What did you, the registrar **S**ee?

What **E**lse did I, the trainer see?

What do you, the registrar **T**hink about this?

What **G**oals can we now set?

What **O**ffers have we got to achieve these goals?

i.e. SETGO.

The method then goes on to suggest these offers are role-played to give the registrar a chance to develop their skills.

This book contains some very useful lists of generic skills necessary to achieve communication goals. They reduce the communication process down to specific behaviours that are practical to teach, i.e. for building rapport:

> ▸ demonstrates good eye contact, posture and movement, facial expression and use of voice techniques (language content, modulation)

- ▸ if the notes or computer are used then it does not interfere with dialogue
- ▸ acknowledges the patients thoughts and feelings non-judgementally
- ▸ expresses concern, understanding, willingness to help and acknowledging the patient's coping efforts
- ▸ deals with sensitive, embarrassing and painful issues sensitively.

The book contains similar lists for all areas of the consultation.

Examination-based methods

One of the major drivers of learning is assessment – particularly if it is either legally essential (summative assessment) or professionally esteemed (MRCGP). It would be foolish for trainers to ignore this motivation – and of course they don't! The Appendix to Chapter 2 contains the current marking schedules for both of these systems and video-based tutorials using these sheets can prove very useful. The trainer and registrar usually mark the consultation and then discuss the presence or absence of the relevant competencies.

Checklist-based methods

These are similar to the exam schedules but are not part of any formal examination process. Details of the those mentioned by trainers are in the appendix to Chapter 2.

Other video-based methods

Body language

Many trainers play the video fast forward with the sound off. This highlights problems with body language to registrars. It tends to look amusing which reduces the threatening element of feedback.

Watching Me, Watching You

This is a video produced by the West Midlands region that provides videos of consultations primarily to help with summative assessment (*see* Appendix to this chapter).

Those Things You Say ...

This is a video-training package produced by the West Midlands Postgraduate General Practice Education Unit in association with the RCGP. It provides a comprehensive guide to the MRCGP Video Assessment of Consulting Skills (*see* Appendix to this chapter).

Sex-lives and Videotape

This is a video produced by the West Midlands Postgraduate General Practice Education Unit. It provides an introduction to sexual health and sexual health history taking. Its target audience is a multi-professional one; thus it is a very good tool for GP registrars to use during their training year.

Homemade movies

Many trainers have kept videos, often of their own consultations, to illustrate certain issues. It seems to de-threaten registrars to show a video 'warts and all' and certainly provides the opportunity for the trainer to show their response to constructive criticism.

John Cleese and Rob Buckman's videos for patients

These are part of a set of training videos that are very amusing and provoke discussion.

Other videos

Some trainers use specific video clips in training. *Dead Poets Society*, starring Robin Williams, has sections that can be used to demonstrate teaching styles and motivation. *Grand Canyon*, starring Kevin Kline, has a section where he is teaching his son to drive, which illustrates the good, the bad and the amazing teaching technique. (I would like to thank Dr Bob Woollard for this pointer.) *See* Chapter 9.

Joint surgeries/visits

This was the second most common method used to assess and teach consulting skills. In Australia, it is the primary teaching method and favoured for its immediacy. It has problems relating to time, the distortion of consultation dynamics and reduction of service time within the practice. Use of Pendleton's rules and role play are useful in a debrief after the consultation (*see* earlier section on Pendleton's rules). Where it does have advantages is in the role modelling demonstration of skills by the trainer and in the opportunity for the trainer to intervene in real time with a real patient. Registrars often comment positively on this and it may be an under-used tool in the UK system. Certainly registrars benefit from sitting in with a range of PHCT (not just other partners) members and seeing a variety of communication styles and techniques. However, this can often be unstructured. Some trainers offer 'filters' to the registrar to help focus them, i.e. 'When sitting in with Dr X concentrate on his connecting or handing over skills' (or whatever, and preferably negotiated with the registrar) and then use these observations as the basis of a tutorial.

Some trainers suggested using Saturday mornings or half-days for this to relieve the time pressure.

Role play

Role play has been mentioned above – it is used commonly by trainers. It can be difficult to introduce with some registrars but many enjoy the fun element of it. It can be a safe way to explore some communication problem areas, i.e. the angry patient, the confrontation, the breaking of bad news. A useful resource in these situations can be a sheet of desirable behaviours that can be referred to and then practised. These instructions can usefully be developed as the initial part of the tutorial between the trainer and the facilitator and then role played with the final backup of the resource sheets. This is the basis of problem-based learning (Barrow and Tamblyn 1980), i.e.:

- ► Problem: the registrar needs to tell someone bad news.
- ► Questions: (generated by the registrar in the tutorial or in preparation).
- ► Solutions: (generated by registrar with facilitation).
- ► Role play of solutions.
- ► Assessment of what works well.
- ► Refer to resource sheet to ensure no major areas missed.
- ► Arrange to look at areas missed (if any) and review use of new skills.

Skills for Communicating with Patients by Silverman *et al.* (1998) has excellent sections covering core skills in all areas of communication, including confrontation and breaking bad news. These make good resource sheets for this sort of exercise.

A particular exercise mentioned for role play was the 'option-raising exercise'. This is useful for the registrar who, often having taken a thorough history considering the patient's agenda well, switches back to a medical doctor-centred model and appears to describe a management plan with no patient involvement. It appears many registrars feel patients expect them to 'behave like a doctor' when it comes to management and they give prescriptive advice. While this may be appropriate on rare occasions, it is one of the areas candidates fail most commonly in the MRCGP video examination component. In this exercise, the trainer role plays a patient (preferably one from the registrar's experience) and the registrar is asked to deliberately discuss *all* the options for management with the trainer. The trainer can use the opportunity to demonstrate the effect patient health beliefs can have on management and help develop negotiation and sharing skills.

Roger Neighbour's *The Inner Consultation* (1987) contains a number of other exercises that can be used in this manner or explored in the consultation itself.

Another exercise mentioned could be described as the RCGP model exercise. The RCGP model simply states that problems have a physical, social and psychological element. Despite the obvious nature of this to GPs, many candidates for the MRCGP do not seem to enquire into this area. If this appears to be a problem, the trainer can role play presentations from the registrar's notes or video using the 'filter' that the registrar must ask some questions that look at these areas. The trainer can try and introduce points that have a bearing on the presentation. This can then be followed by a discussion on how this would influence the consultation for both the doctor and the patient (*see* BATHE exercise in Chapter 13).

Tutorial-based exercises

A number of these were mentioned by trainers. Generally they are methods that tackle particular problems that have emerged with registrars, and are done in pairs with the trainer.

Listening skills exercise

This is useful where there is evidence that the registrar is perhaps interrupting or not listening to the patient. The registrar is asked to describe a particular event (i.e. most useful learning experience, best holiday, etc.) and the trainer demonstrates 'active listening'. There is then a discussion where the learner identifies the components of active listening and the roles are reversed. A variant is for the trainer to deliberately demonstrate the opposite skills (destructive listening?). The trainer then summarises by reinforcing the relevant skills. The whole process can be video-taped to allow better review.

Empathic language exercise

This is useful where the registrar appears to be using personal language constructs inappropriately with patients (often very medicalised complex language). This probably impedes development of rapport. The registrar is asked to describe an event that has some emotional content for them for two to three minutes. The trainer summarises this twice: first, using different words and with interpretation, and second, using the registrar's language content and reflection. After a discussion about how this felt for the registrar, the trainer describes a similar event and the registrar summarises this using the trainer's language and reflection. The trainer then reinforces the new skills demonstrated.

Many more of these type of exercises are described in Philip Burnard's *Teaching Interpersonal Skills* (*see* Chapter 10).

Assessing consultation skills and needs

The summative type of assessment, needs assessment and teaching of consultation skills often seem to be bound up in the same teaching situation. This is not necessarily a problem but it does create the potential for confusion. Somewhere in the teaching process there needs to be an acknowledgement of this, so an attempt to find any 'blind spots' is made. How did trainers tackle this? A number of processes seemed to be employed:

▶ Use of the examination marking schedules.
▶ Use of process type models that include the patient agenda.
▶ Use of other consultation maps/skill checklists.
▶ The 'gut-weighted approach', i.e. the trainer feels *comfortable* with the registrar's consultations and has had no worrying feedback. The registrar seems to be enjoying the process 'energetically' as one trainer put it.

These are all described in the Appendix to this chapter. The most significant feature would seem to be recognition of the potential problem in this area.

Summary comments

There is an interesting dichotomy between the type of teaching method that uses an intuitive process and that using a logical process. Some would say this relates to the hemispheric cerebral dominance inherent in the assessor, i.e. you are left dominant so logical, rational and controlled (the scientist), or right dominant and creative, intuitive and spontaneous (the artist). Both approaches have value that needs to be acknowledged and it is probably a mistake to use either exclusively. This chapter offers practical approaches for consultation skills teaching for each of your cerebral hemispheres and some that may even involve both!

Appendix to Chapter 4

Consultation mapping (from Pendleton et al. 1984)

This process makes the assumption that every consultation should include a number of defined activities and that these usually progress in a logical order. Many trainers feel that these assumptions are not always valid. Nevertheless, mapping can help a registrar with a disorganised approach to the consultation.

A video is watched and the particular activity occurring as the doctor speaks or at minute intervals is recorded on the forms with a mark by both registrar and trainer.

Activity	Time elapsed in consultation (mins)
	1 2 3 4 5 6 7 8 9 10 11 12

1 Opening the consultation
2 Nature and history of problem
3 Aetiology of problem
4 Patient's ideas
5 Patient's expectations
6 Patient's concerns
7 Effects of problem
8 Continuing problems
9 At risk factors
10 Action taken
11 Sharing understanding
12 Involving in management
13 Closing the consultation

These stages are sometimes represented on a line chart that can be seen to imply the line should progress 'smoothly' from the left to right.

Neurolinguistic programming – language systems: visual, auditory and kinaesthetic (VAK)

VAK preference indicator (from Rose 1985 *Accelerated Learning*)

This gives a score to indicate your VAK preferences. Circle the response that you would feel appropriate for you in most cases.

When you:

spell, do you	try to see the word?	use phonetic approaches?	write it down to see if it 'feels' right?
visualise, do you	see vivid pictures?	think in sounds?	have few images that usually involve movement?
concentrate, do you	find visual images distracting?	find sounds distracting?	find movement distracting?
are angry, do you	go quiet and seethe?	have a verbal outburst?	storm off, grit your teeth and smash something?
forget something, do you	forget names but not faces?	forget faces but not names?	remember mostly what you wanted to do?

contact someone (work-related), do you	prefer face-to-face?	prefer the phone?	prefer to do something with them (golf, walk)?
are relaxing, do you	prefer to watch TV, cinema, a play?	listen to music or the radio?	walk, play sport or play games?
are interpreting someone's mood, do you?	look at their face?	listen to their tone of voice?	watch their body language?
reward someone, do you	write them a note?	give them oral praise?	give them a hug/pat?
are inactive, do you	look about, watch something, doodle?	talk to yourself or others?	fidget?
are talking, do you	talk and listen sparingly?	enjoy listening but want to talk?	use gestures a lot?
are learning, do you	like posters, slides, diagrams, etc.?	like talks, talking, verbal cues?	prefer activity, i.e. role play, 'doing'?
TOTAL	V	A	K

Physical characteristics

	V	A	K
Face	• Eyes move first • Blinks a lot • Looks up to think • Eyes steady when looking • Looks at people • Little facial expression	• Mumbles when thinking and reading • Closes eyes often • Listens intently • Nods to sounds often • Looks sideways thinking	• Eyes move randomly • Looks down to think • Doesn't need to look at people or path • Uses expressions and gestures
Gestures	• Small and precise • Neat and orderly • Little use of touch • Few gestures	• Rhythmic and repetitive • Counts on fingers • Strokes • More gestures when talking	• BIG gestures • Likes to touch and hold things • Lots of gestures • Points at things
Body	• Still and slow • Erect posture • Stands or sits away • Looks before moving	• Sways or rocks • Leans towards things	• Erratic, clumsy • Sits close or on • Moves a lot • Exaggerated movements
Voice	• Quiet and quick • Long sentences • Few pauses • Precise	• Rhythmic • Song-like quality • Repeats message • Mimics tone, pitch, etc.	• Slow and slurred • Sounds more than words • Short sentences

Language

	V	A	K
Nouns	light, eye, vision, colours, pictures, views, scenes, flashes, sights, spaces, perspective	mouth, bell, tongue, speech, talk, voices, notes, tales, words, hearing, ears, sound, noise	feelings, touch, calm, mind, control, panic, pressure, hold, connection
Verbs	to see, to visualise, to appear, to image, to picture, to look	to hear, to listen, to express, to ring, to describe, to voice	to touch, to feel, to come to grips, to control, to hold
Adjectives	hazy, dim, bright	unheard of, dull, quiet, noisy	sharp, blunt, hot, cool, stiff, loose

These words can give an indication of the learner's and facilitator's preferred systems. It may be possible to use this concept in teaching and it certainly raises the awareness of the value of language both in education and the consultation.

Behavioural preferences

	V	A	K
Learning	• Likes colours, pictures, patterns • Wants a model to copy • Likes to read	• Likes to talk and listen • Wants to verbally rephrase learning	• Likes to do • Likes to enjoy • Likes 'hands on' • Is a creative thinker

Memory	• Visual memory	• Auditory memory going over	• Remembers by 'doing'
Praise	• Likes visible praise, 'look at this you did'	• Likes auditory praise, 'well done'	• Likes physical praise – pat on back
Environs	• Likes quietness, neatness and stillness	• Distracted by sounds • Likes groups	• Works well 1:1
Listening	• Mind wanders quickly • Wants quick, precise, verbal instructions	• Likes stepwise instruction and to repeat this back	• Likes speech and action linked
Planning	• Plans ahead in their mind, 'seeing' the goal	• Plans step by step, ticking them off	• Tends not to plan but will review
Dress	• Neat, precise, coordinated • Bright and colourful	• Dresses in 'harmony' • Often in fashion	• Wears what feels good – often loose

The value of this list may be in recognising behavioural preferences and matching teaching styles to them where possible.

Examination-based methods of video assessment

The marking schedules for summative assessment and the MRCGP video assessment are shown below. Details of precisely how they are used in these two examinations are not included. Some of the criteria are difficult to define and will be open to interpretation. Discussing them with one of the assessors or examiners can help – but not always, as the definitions seem elusive!

SUMMATIVE ASSESSMENT VIDEO MARKING CRITERIA

Major error/s seen?
Minor error/s seen?

Listening:	1	2	3	4	5	6
Action:	1	2	3	4	5	6
Understanding:	1	2	3	4	5	6

Challenge: Low Medium High

Assessment: Refer Pass
      Clear refer Clear pass

Rating scale: 1 refer
     2 probably refer
     3 bare pass
     4 competent
     5 good
     6 excellent

Listening: identifies and elucidates reason for attendance. An acceptable plan should be negotiated.
Action: appropriate action to identify patients problem.

Reasonable referral/investigation. Help sought when necessary. Management appropriate.

Understanding: registrar understands process/outcome of consultation. Action explained. Obvious shortcomings identified and relevant background mentioned.

Errors: single major error or series of minor errors leads to referral. Major error defined as causing actual or potential harm. Minor error causes inconvenience only.

Challenge refers to the registrar's perception of the difficulty of the consultation.

MRCGP video-marking schedule

The MRCGP video-marking schedule is based on a defined series of competencies that should be demonstrated. These are marked present if a certain performance criterion (PC) is judged to be demonstrated. Not all the competencies are included in the marking schedule but more are likely to creep in over the years. The list below contains all the competencies and highlights those currently (1998) in the marking schedule.

* Indicates currently in marking schedule.
** Indicates currently used to assess for merit.

DISCOVER THE REASON FOR ATTENDANCE

A Elicit the patient's account of the symptoms which made him or her come to the doctor:
* PC   the doctor encourages the patient's contribution at appropriate points
* PC   the doctor responds to cues.

B Obtain the relevant items of social and occupational circumstances:
* PC   appropriate details are obtained to place the complaints in a social and psychological context
 PC   the doctor is able to establish the effect of the illness on work or home life.

C Explore the patient's health understanding:
** PC the patient's health understanding is taken into account in enough detail to ensure there is a reasonable probability the consultation will be successful.

D Enquire about continuing problems:

PC   information obtained allows an assessment
        on whether a continuing complaint represents
        an issue which must be addressed in this
        consultation.

DEFINE THE CLINICAL PROBLEM(S)

A Obtain additional information about symptoms
and details of medical history:

* PC   sufficient information is obtained for no
        serious condition to be missed

PC   verbal investigation is consistent with the
        hypothesis which could reasonably have been
        formed: the doctor appears open to more than
        one explanation of the problem.

B Assess the condition of the patient by physical
inspection if appropriate:

* PC   the examination chosen is likely to confirm or
        disprove hypotheses which could reasonably
        have been formed *or* is designed to address a
        patient's concern.

C Making a working diagnosis:

* PC   the doctor appears to make a clinically appro-
        priate working diagnosis.

EXPLAIN THE PROBLEM(S) TO THE
PATIENT

A Share the findings with the patient:

* PC   diagnosis, management and effects of treat-
        ment are explained.

B Tailor the explanation to the patient:
* PC   content and language chosen are appropriate to what the patient needs
** PC explanation utilises (without necessarily adopting) some or all of the patient's elicited beliefs.

C Ensure that the explanation is understood and accepted by the patient:
** PC efforts are made to confirm the patients understanding and an attempt is made to reconcile the doctors viewpoint with that of the patient.

ADDRESS THE PATIENT'S PROBLEM

A Assess the severity of the presenting problem(s):
PC   problems of differing severity are differentiated and treated with the correct weight.

B Choose an appropriate form of management:
* PC   the management is appropriate for the working diagnosis and reflects a good understanding of modern accepted medical practice.

C Involve the patient in the management plan to an appropriate degree:
* PC   management options are shared with the patient.

MAKE EFFECTIVE USE OF THE CONSULTATION

A Make efficient use of resources:
PC   the doctor makes sensible use of available time and suggests further consultation as appropriate

PC   investigations ordered are capable of con-
        firming or excluding the working diagnosis
        and the costs are justified in terms of the
        refinements the results might make to the
        overall management of the case
PC   other health professionals are considered and
        involved appropriately (or not)
★ PC   the doctor's prescribing behaviour is appro-
        priate.

B Establish a relationship with the patient:
★ PC   allowing for the nature of the consultation the
        patient and the doctor appear to have estab-
        lished rapport *or* the doctor understands why
        no rapport has been established.

C Give opportunistic health promotion advice:
PC   at-risk factors are dealt with appropriately in
        the consultation.

More details on the MRCGP process are provided in
Chapter 7.

Other checklist resources for looking at videos

The summative assessment process and MRCGP have sidelined checklist methods used in the past. This may be a shame because these were developed with learning in mind and not from a purely assessment point of view. Five of these scales are shown below and some trainers find this approach more useful than the exam-based one. Registrars, however, are conscious of the hoops they now have to jump through so the use of these scales needs some introduction. They can be useful to highlight particular areas of need in individual registrars.

Ten-task consultation numeric analogue scale

The consultation observed (video or sitting in) is graded 1–6 against a number of tasks. This is done openly and with discussion.

Scale: 1 = perfect, through to 6 = not seen.

Task	Scale 1–6	Positive comments	Recommendations
1 The doctor's greeting (verbal and non-verbal) was helpful to the patient			
2 The doctor defined the reason for attendance			
3 The doctor elicited the patient's ideas, concerns and expectations			
4 The doctor considered continuing and at-risk factors			
5 The doctor encouraged the patient to participate in decision making			

Task	Scale 1–6	Positive comments	Recommendations
6 The doctor offered appropriate follow-up			
7 The doctor tried to modify health-seeking behaviour appropriately			
8 The doctor used resources well (time, referral, PHCT, etc.)			
9 The doctor responded to cues			
10 The doctor used appropriate skills when information giving			

This sort of numeric analogue scale might suit the more 'logical' thinker (trainer or registrar).

37-task consultation visual analogue scale

A similar scale was described in the *BMJ* some years ago. It is an analogue scale of 37 elements so is considerably more detailed and could be used to tease out some more areas for teaching, perhaps for the registrar who has good communication skills and would like a more in-depth approach. In practice, most trainers find 10 or so areas plenty. It is worth bearing in mind the old adage that the human mind can only hold between four and seven points on a particular area at one time, so perhaps 10 is even stretching things! The scale might also be attractive to those with a strong analytical approach.

For those interested the reference is *BMJ* **306**: 1044 (1993).

11-task consultation visual analogue scale

This scale contains many of the previous elements but uses a visual presentation style that might suit those with the NLP 'visual' programme (*see* Appendix to Chapter 2)

The registrar and trainer evaluate the consultation by placing a mark that reflects his or her view on a line between the two polarising statements.

1 Nature and history of problems fully defined	Nature and history of problems poorly defined
2 Aetiology of problems fully defined	Aetiology of problems not defined at all
3 Patient's ideas, concerns and expectations fully explored	Patients ideas, concerns and expectations unexplored
4 Effects of problems fully considered	Effects of problems ignored
5 Continuing problems fully considered	Continuing problems ignored
6 At-risk factors considered	At-risk factors ignored

7 Appropriate action chosen for each problem	————	Inappropriate actions taken for problems
8 Doctor shares understanding	————	No evidence of sharing understanding
9 Patient involved in management	————	Patient not involved in management
10 Resources are used well	————	Resources are used poorly
11 A good relationship is established with the patient	————	Unhelpful/ deteriorating relationship with the patient

This will highlight areas for discussion.

The UBC evaluation scale (from the UBC Residents Handbook)

This form seems to include useful detail that could be helpful in specific situations, i.e. to bring out para-language features, problem solving skills, etc.

AREA OBSERVED	COMMENT
Communication	
► registrar appearance, behaviour	
► listening skills	

- paralanguage features (speech rate, pause/speech ratio, tone, volume, clarity, articulation)
- word choice, sentence structure
- logic (orderly, complicated, ambivalent, magical)
- response to patient's 'private' language

Self-awareness
- feelings, personal emotions, behaviour
- transference, countertransference

Clinical problem solving
- cue detection
- efficiency of questions
- probability ranking
- management plan
- evidence base
- consideration of alternatives
- involvement of patient

Doctor/patient
- establishing rapport – 'hearing' the story
- doctor/patient-centredness
- incorporation of patient's perception in explanation
- encouragement of patient's understanding/involvement
- empathy
- attitude
- ethical considerations

Efficiency
- organisation
- time management, including screening behaviour
- closure skills
- use of examination

Consultation task judgemental scale

Some trainers described using a task-orientated scale with a marking grid using terms that range from 'unacceptable' to 'very good'. This seems very judgemental in nature and does not seem to have any advantages over the analogue or exam-based scales. The assessment of whether behaviour is not quite acceptable or acceptable seems very arbitrary and has the potential to alienate the learner. This scale is not reproduced here for that reason.

Video-training packages

- *Watching Me, Watching You*: a video-training package including a comprehensive workbook to support the summative assessment process.
- *Those Things You Say ...*: a video-training package and comprehensive workbook to support MRCGP Video Assessment of Consulting Skills.
- *Sex-lives and Videotape*: a video-training package. This is a multi-professional learning tool, very useful for GP registrars.

All of these packages can be obtained from Radcliffe Medical Press. Tel: 01235 528820 or www.radcliffe-oxford.com

CHAPTER 5

Curriculum-based resources: how do trainers define a curriculum?

How do I know what I need to know?

The unconscious incompetent

Introduction

Perhaps the questions should be '*do* trainers need to define a curriculum?' and '*how* do trainers decide on the *core* of knowledge, skills and attitudes that should be acquired by the registrar?'. Two main approaches to the problem seem to exist: first the *objectives* approach and second the *experiential* or *process* approach.

The objective approach to curricular planning sets objectives that are specific enough for assessment without being voluminous and unusable. The problem is often that the objectives change in time, place and person (not all objectives are relevant to all registrars). This approach is epitomised by the following quotation:

Education must have an end in view for it is not an end in itself.

Marshall

The experiential/process approach views the development of the registrar as a transformation from undifferentiated doctor to GP. The process involves reflection on experience to develop learning needs. Fostering a set of beliefs and values is the prime task. Of course, by its very nature, this is harder to define and assess. The Dean of St Paul's Cathedral illustrates this philosophy in this quotation:

> The aim of education is the knowledge not of fact but of values.

Inge

Whichever philosophy one adopts, Guilbert (1997) has described the four 'Cs' of curriculum development that seem both practical and valid:

► Cooperation: the curriculum requires the input of both learners, teachers and the people who do the job – preferably groups of all three.
► Continuous: the curriculum needs to evolve continuously.
► Comprehensive: the curriculum needs to be a tool that helps direct learners when devising their learning goals. It needs to point towards all the important areas.
► Concrete: the curriculum needs to be specific so that learners can tell in which direction it is pointing. This does not contradict the continuous evolution of the curriculum but infers a well-defined set of objectives.

The WONCA Educational Meeting (Fabb 1997) suggested the following five-step process to help devise curricular statements:

1 Define the roles and tasks of the doctor within the setting.
2 Determine the required values, attitudes, skills and knowledge.
3 Clarify what needs to be done to acquire these attributes.
4 Determine how the trainer can assist in this process.
5 Determine how the registrar will know when that has been achieved.

This chapter describes how trainers are dealing with this difficult area. There is a degree of overlap with Chapter 1 that is indicated in the text.

Objectives-related methods of curriculum development

Wolverhampton Grid	Combined confidence rating scale	Initial educational planning list
Manchester rating scales	Dartford rating scales	Regional documentation
SA trainers report		

Learner-centred confidence rating scales

Many of the needs assessment tools described in Chapter 1 are based on the concept of a core curriculum. The fact that they all vary shows how elusive this core is! Details on the lists mentioned are available in either the Appendix to Chapter 1 or Appendix A, as indicated.

Wolverhampton Grid (*see* Appendix A)

This is a long and potentially daunting document. However, it covers a wide spectrum of general practice and was commonly mentioned by trainers.

Combined confidence rating scale (*see* Appendix A)

This is a scale collated from a number of locally generated lists that seems to cover many areas particularly well and succinctly.

Initial educational planning list

This scale really checks the basics that some would argue should have been covered prior to the training year. In practice it seems to highlight at least two or three needs in most registrars that can be quite a surprise (*see* Appendix A).

Teacher-centred rating scales

These scales are designed to be scored by the trainer after observation and feedback about the registrar. They are often used more openly and rated either jointly or by the registrar directly. They are based on a defined set of desirable attributes inherent in the scale.

Manchester rating scales (*see* Appendix A)

This lengthy occasional paper was used in two main ways: to browse through or to use in small sections where thought relevant. It does attempt to be inclusive and cover all the main areas so could provide a tool to highlight blindspots if necessary.

Dartford rating scales

These scales are perhaps similar in approach to the Manchester rating scales but are more user-friendly. Some of these are reproduced in the appendix to this chapter and cover the following areas:

► relationship with patients and relatives
► history taking and interviewing scales
► physical examination
► use of investigations
► problem solving
► implementation of management plan.

Deanery documentation

Many deaneries produce formative assessment packages that contain rating scales of various types – many with a curricular feel to them. Most do not attempt to be detailed but do offer useful 'umbrella'-type coverage.

The trainer's report

This is essentially an objectives-based curriculum document. Advice on its use in training is covered in Chapter 8.

Attribute definition methods

JCGPT list	RCGP Occasional Paper 30	The Future GP
A–Z list	RCGP Occasional Paper 4	RACGP list
Specific lists		

Some bodies have attempted to define the desirable attributes, skills and abilities a GP should possess. Others have tried to break this down into educational aims. Some examples are described below.

JCGPT *Training for General Practice* (1992)

This publication contains the following statements:

Values and attributes

Fully trained GPs are expected to be:

1 caring and understanding of patients and families
2 committed to high-quality care
3 aware of the need to be readily accessible and available

4 aware of their own limitations and willing to seek help from others when appropriate

5 committed to keeping up to date both clinically and organisationally

6 committed to improving the quality of their professional performance through active participation in quality assurance and audit

7 aware of and committed to observing the ethical principles that govern the medical profession

8 appreciative of the value of teamwork to patient care in general practice

9 willing to teach others, including the wider PHCT, and willing to acquire the skills to achieve this

10 willing to contribute to the advancement of medical knowledge when possible

11 able to care for themselves and to achieve a balance between personal and professional life.

Clinical competence

General practitioners are expected to be:

1 knowledgeable about general practice. (including an understanding of the physical psychological, behavioural, epidemiological, social, disease-based and scientific aspects of medicine)

2 skilled in recognising and making appropriate decisions about every problem presented to them by patients

3 able to examine a patient's physical and mental state and to use investigations appropriately

4 able to assess symptoms and physical signs, to establish a diagnosis when possible and to exercise sound judgement in further management

5 skilled in the process of communication. This will involve the ability to listen and to explain carefully and effectively to patients, their families and others. It will

include the ability to involve patients in management decisions

6 able to contribute to the prevention and promotion of health both personally and within the context of the PHCT and society

7 able and willing to deal with appropriate emergencies

8 able to prescribe effectively with regard to the effects of over- and under-prescribing

9 able to keep clear, coherent, up-to-date records suitable for clinical and audit use.

Organisational ability

General practitioners are expected to be:

1 able to assess health status, needs and expectations of practice populations

2 able to plan, organise and manage a practice to provide the range of accessible services (acute and chronic illness, emergencies, health promotion)

3 able to function as a member of a team and adopt the appropriate team role, including leader where appropriate. This involves an understanding of the roles, skills and responsibilities of each member of the PHCT

4 able to make effective use of resources (money, time, skill-mix) within and outside the practice setting

5 able to organise and carry out effective clinical audit (including the management of change)

6 conversant with and willing to participate in the work of organisations that advise, plan and assist the development of health-related services and healthcare professions.

Comment: this list makes interesting reading and may be helpful for the registrar and trainer to develop educational aims. It could certainly be used in parts to form the basis of discussion in a tutorial. However, it leaves many areas poorly defined.

Curricular aims method

These methods list a set of desirable abilities, attributes and values or goals, which can be used to help define learning objectives. Each of these lists is different – some seem too long to be practically useful, others too non-specific to be applicable. Each of them seems to have selective value, provide an overview that can limit blindspots and stimulate some interesting discussion and thought.

The Oxford Deaneries Course Organisers and Advisers Group list

This is published as Occasional paper No. 30 by the RCGP and contains a comprehensive list of objectives. This list covers:

▶ patient care
▶ communication
▶ organisation
▶ professional values
▶ personal and professional growth.

The authors claim that the list is valid, important, attainable and assessable.

The Future General Practitioner: learning and teaching

This book by Fry (1972) contains a lot of useful information despite its age. It includes a list of 11 goals for GPs that seem very relevant today:

1 ability to make diagnoses which are expressed in physical, psychological and social terms simultaneously
2 recognition of the patient as a unique individual can modify the ways in which they elicit data, make hypotheses and manage illness

3 the ability to make appropriate decisions about every presented problem

4 understanding of the way interpersonal relationships can affect the way illness occurs, presents and responds to treatment

5 ability to understand and manage the use of time-scale in a manner peculiar to general practice

6 have knowledge of and skills in using the wide range of possible interventions

7 understanding of the relationship between health and illness and the social characteristics of the patient

8 have knowledge of and skills in practice management

9 have recognition of the need for CME

10 have an understanding of basic research methods in practice

11 demonstrate ability and willingness to be self-critical (including audit).

A system of training for General Practice

The Exeter University Department of General Practice produced *A system of training for general practice* (Pereira Gray 1979), which contains the following list of desired abilities in a registrar:

1 knows what it feels like to be a patient

2 maintains the dignity of patients at all times

3 practises patient-centred medicine

4 identifies his or her own learning needs

5 remedies his or her own learning needs

6 assesses himself or herself objectively

7 accurately analyses his or her doctor/patient relationships

8 understands illness as deeply in terms of the patient's behaviour as in pathological terms

9 assesses accurately the capacity of a home/household to care for a sick member

10 offers (in more than 50% of cases) practical preventative advice

11 can tolerate uncertainty

12 promotes patient autonomy

13 reads and critically analyses the literature of GP

14 regards GP as a branch of medicine with its own set of skills, attitudes and knowledge

15 feels a responsibility for the health of his or her registered population generally

16 can analyse a problem, devise a research project, carry this out and present the results.

This is published as RCGP Occasional Paper No. 4.

The A–Z list

This is an approach that tries to define the outcome aims against a curricular structure. It covers the following areas:

- Introductory course
- Audit/research
- Child health
- Chronic disease management
- Common symptoms
- Complementary medicine
- Consultation
- Dermatology
- ENT
- Ethics
- Eyes
- Family planning
- Finances
- Gynaecology
- Infectious disease/immunity
- MRCGP
- Obstetrics
- Organisation
- Personal/professional growth

- ► Psychiatry
- ► Rheumatology/orthopaedics
- ► Screening
- ► Substance abuse
- ► Surgical skills
- ► Teams
- ► Terminal care
- ► Therapeutics.

The list is extensive but not exhaustive and the aims are not designed to be all inclusive. They are an offer on which to base and/or check the development of the learning process. The full aims under each category are listed in the Appendix to this chapter.

The Royal Australian College of General Practice (RACGP) list

This is a list of 23 goals for registrars to aim at contained in the book *Focus on Learning* (Fabb *et al.* 1976). This book contains a lot of educational material and the list makes interesting reading but probably adds little to the sum of the others mentioned above.

Specific area lists

Difficult list	Ethics and law list	Need to know list
Forms you should know list	GMC lists	IT list

These lists provide specific structure in certain areas. They have the potential to produce a very teacher-centred approach unless balanced by a learner-based needs assessment process, i.e. in normal language, if the learner has needs in these areas the list may help. Details are provided in Appendix A.

The 'difficult' list

This list arose out of a joint trainer/registrar session. It includes areas many registrars have difficulty with early on in the year. It helps to highlight these areas and legitimise help-seeking behaviour in the registrar.

'Forms you should know' list

This is a simple checklist of the relevant documentation designed to raise awareness.

Ethics and law list

A simple list of areas to be considered (*see* Appendix to this chapter).

The 'need to know' list

A list attempting to prioritise learning needs at the start of the year. It is primarily pragmatic and administrative.

BMA guidance

The BMA produces guidance booklets on many areas (minor surgery, out-of-hours recommendations, innovative VTS schemes) that make interesting reading and can be obtained free from the BMA.

The IT list

The NHS executive has produced a list of computer skills for training practices (*see* Appendix to this chapter).

Process-related methods of curriculum development

A number of tools for facilitating this process were mentioned by trainers.

Reflective learning

This is a process widely accepted as a major tool to enhance learning. So what is it? Essentially it involves systems designed to raise awareness of the learning opportunities generated by experience. It has been defined as 'a dialogue of thinking and doing through which I become more skilful' (Schon 1987). In practice, most of these opportunities fly by and are lost in the 'heat of battle'. Al-Shehri (1995; *see* Chapter 10) discusses refinements of a number of tools that many trainers already use in this area. These can be divided into a number of areas:

Recording experiences

Many experiences will be remembered and raised by most registrars but will still tend to be only a minority of cases. The value of this system is to open up many more experiences to the learning process. Three main methods of recording exist:

- The log: this is a simple record of events that lacks much personal input. It is easier to produce but less useful as a result.
- The diary: this encourages the learner to record feelings/interpretations.
- The journal: this combines the other two approaches but requires time input.

Trainers' experience suggests it is difficult to get many registrars to record a lot of detail. It is perhaps expecting too much at a time when they are bombarded with a multitude of demands. However, the following tips seem to help:

- buy them a diary
- keep one yourself and demonstrate its use (get your partners involved too)
- look at both diaries together regularly
- start by asking them questions. Write these in the diary, i.e. when sitting in with a partner you could write: What do they do best? How could you learn to do it? What did they do that surprised you?
- give them 'filters' and write these in the diary, i.e. This week record the situations that make you feel angry (if anger seems to be a problem). It can be used to boost confidence (write down when a patient gave you positive feedback, write down when you did something right, etc.) and to look at any other area of need.

Giving feedback

Al-Shehri (1995) suggests the level of feedback needs to be matched to the cognition level of the registrar. This is judged by the way the registrar reports their experience. Al-Shehri describes five levels of cognition with corresponding appropriate levels for reflective feedback. These are shown in Table 5.1.

Table 5.1: Feedback matched to level of cognition and reflection

Cognitive ability	Level of reflection	Feedback
Level 1 Receiving knowledge	Receiving experience	Relating knowledge/ experience Trying to look at understanding
Level 2 Comprehension and responding	Describing experience	Looking at what happened Trying to look at meaning
Level 3 Application/valuing	Extracting meaning	Looking at quality issues Opening methods for analysis
Level 4 Analysis	Analysing experience	Comparing/classifying Introducing idea of principles
Level 5 Synthesis/extrapolation	Combining elements	Summarising/theorising

Some of this seems to have limited practical value but a number of principles seem to emerge to aid the giving of feedback:

► base the feedback at the level of the reflection – try and move it up to the next level
► each feedback needs an element of support and encouragement
► the process needs to be continuous.

A number of types of diary user seem to emerge. The 'descriptor' writes a bland list of what happened. The 'analyst' breaks down the reasons behind events.

The 'evaluator' does both of these tasks but also looks at the personal and professional implications. The trainer can try and influence which of these types the registrar adopts to suit the educational agenda. The cycle in Figure 5.1 summarises the reflective learning cycle. Often it is helpful to make the process explicit to the registrar and in this instance even a little bit of educational theory seems helpful.

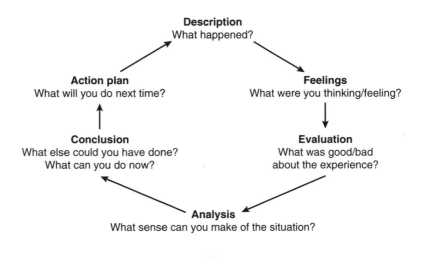

Figure 5.1: The reflective learning cycle (Kolb 1974).

Self-directed learning

It is difficult to find a succinct definition of self-directed learning. Basically it is a learner-centred process that encourages the registrar to discover and define his or her own learning needs, explore his or her own learning methods and evaluate his or her own development, with facilitation as required.

So when is this appropriate? Guglielmo (in Fabb *et al.* 1976) identified seven factors associated with successful self-directed learning outcomes:

1 High openness to learning, dominated by enjoyment and enthusiasm. Independent, strongly motivated learners.
2 Good self-concept as a learner – organised learners with good problem solving and reading skills. Confident working alone with self-discipline.
3 High initiative and independence – one of the characteristics of poor learning is learners who restrict themselves to tasks defined by outside influences (i.e. summative assessment) and look forward to the end of the learning process.
4 High enjoyment of verbal discussion with a belief in the exploratory nature of education.
5 An integrative approach where new ideas are related to the existing framework.
6 A drive to self-improvement and achievement.
7 An acceptance of responsibility for one's own learning.

These principles can be assessed by the self-directed learning readiness scale (SDLRS), which is a validated tool that has been applied in general practice. Details of this scale can be found in an article by Bligh (1992).

Total quality management (TQM) and the pursuit of excellence

TQM is a management tool developed to maximise efficiency. Its basic tenet is that everyone in a system should strive to exceed expectations by maximising the use of every resource at every level. Can trainers provide TQE (total quality education)? What are the hallmarks of the 'excellent' educational product? A list of the 14 hallmarks of excellence in registrars is contained in Neighbour's (1992) *The Inner Apprentice* (*see* Chapter 11). These may point trainers in the direction of TQE and are shown in Box 5.1.

The challenging questions are 'Are these teachable and how?' and 'Which ones can I teach and how?'. Some of the tools in this manual address these points.

Box 5.1: The 14 hallmarks of excellence in registrars

Positive response to novelty
Genuine caring with respect for people
Good clinical competence
Good self-awareness
Good group skills
Good personal qualities (undefined)
High educability (undefined)
Strong motivation
A balanced lifestyle/personality
Industrious
Good communication skills
A sense of mission
Good critical abilities
Good diversity of approach

Problem-based learning (Barrow and Tamblyn 1980)

This technique is being used in several undergraduate teaching programmes and has been described by many authors. Essentially, the learner identifies what problems they face in their working environment, develops learning needs based on these observations and then plans how to meet these needs. Finally the objectives are tested back in the problem setting. The trainer's role is to oversee the process, advise on resources when asked and ultimately assess the validity of the final objectives reached, that is:

▶ The registrar realises he or she is having problems with skin diagnoses.
▶ The registrar develops the following needs:
  – need for a structured diagnostic approach
  – need for a better knowledge base
  – need for feedback on outcomes.
▶ The registrar decides:
  – to ask which book the trainer recommends and why?
  – to have two tutorials based on the registrar's patients with the partner who possesses the Dip. Derm.
  – to routinely clinically review all dermatological cases
  – to reassess the situation in six weeks
  – to discuss the solutions with the trainer in six weeks.

It appears that groups of four to six learners will identify all the major learning objectives in a given situation that were agreed by a group of experienced doctors. (Coulson and Osbourne 1984). However, the application of pure problem-based learning in the 1:1 setting has not been studied. Registrars in this setting are likely to need guidance in setting learning goals. The concept does encourage trainers to adopt a more learner-centred style.

Summary comments

An interesting idea in the concept of curricular development comes from the Royal Australian College of General Practice (RACGP) – the 'three-dimensional approach to family medicine education'. This describes the content of three axes that encapsulate the curriculum of family medicine. These are described below.

The competent GP requires:

Axis 1: A set of values, skills, knowledge and attitudes

1 values and attitudes
2 interpersonal and communication skills
3 problem solving skills
4 interpretative skills
5 perceptual and manual skills
6 recall/access to facts.

Axis 2: Clinical competencies

1 understanding the individual, family and community
2 analysing and defining health problems
3 managing health problems
4 adopting a promotive and preventative approach
5 accepting the appropriate responsibility.

Axis 3: Skills in managing the spectrum of clinical and managerial problems in practice

1 managing the full age range – neonate to very old patient (neonate, infant, toddler, schoolchild, adolescent, young adult, pregnancy, middle age, early old age, late old age)
2 using skills and knowledge from a variety of disciplines
3 applying various theories in problem assessment/ management (systems, analytical, etc.)
4 applying a knowledge of family dynamics
5 applying management skills.

It seems apparent that every trainer uses a variety of methods in developing the concept of the curriculum. Some of these appear concrete, some much more abstract.

The following guidelines have been offered on this subject that seem to combine these two approaches (WONCA conference booklet 1997):

► Try and agree on the basic values that underpin the discipline of practice in your health system.

► Define the attitudes, skills, values and knowledge for a small number of competencies that are essential for professional performance to the appropriate standard.

► Create a curriculum that is learner-orientated, problem-based, competency-focused, patient-orientated and community-centred.

► Ensure the curriculum embodies the principles of adult learning.

► Develop a set of curricular objectives balanced by a curricular process.

► Use the five-step process (*see* Introduction to Chapter 3) (define the roles and tasks/determine the necessary values, attitudes, knowledge and skills/clarify how to achieve these/determine how the trainer can help/work out how you will know they have been achieved).

► Look at the 3D model to ensure all aspects have been considered.

► Use the whole process for both planning and assessment.

► Provide the learning opportunities within the practising environment and surround the learner with good role models.

It has been asked 'On what is the curriculum based if it is not centred on the student?' and many trainers find they evolve from the concrete type of curriculum to the abstract evolutionary model. This is illustrated in Figure 5.2.

It has been suggested that the trainer needs to evolve from a content-based approach before the process-based model can function adequately. Whether you are an abstractive process-orientated or concrete content-based trainer this section offers some tools that can be useful in curriculum development.

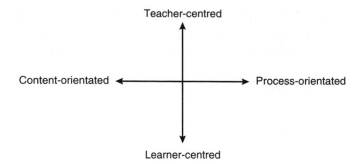

Questions
- Where did you start?
- Where are you now?
- Where do you want to be?

▼

Figure 5.2: Curriculum orientation.

Appendix to Chapter 5

Dartford rating scales

These scales are rated by the trainer using the following grid:

1 **Inadequate**	many major deficiencies in this area performs conspicuously below the standard you would expect from their peers
2 **Marginal**	important deficiencies in this area performs less well than most of their peers
3 **Proficient**	few deficiencies of significance performs as well as most of peer group
4	
5 **Superior**	generally impressive and well above average

Six of these scales are printed after this introduction. Further details can be obtained from Dr Norton Short, Course Organiser, Dartford VTS.

Aspect A

Relationships with patient and family

This aspect is concerned with the registrar's willingness and ability to establish an effective relationship with the patient (and family where appropriate).

Ineffective		*Effective*	*Not appraised*
1 Gruff or cold in approach	1 2 3 4 5	Establishes a comfortable and professional rapport	0
2 Lacks tact and discretion	1 2 3 4 5	Tactful and discreet in discussion	0
3 Exhibits a subtle disapproval of certain patients	1 2 3 4 5	Accepts patients' history and behaviour as they are	0
4 Becomes overinvolved	1 2 3 4 5	Does not become overinvolved	0
5 Discourages patients from expressing their thoughts and fears	1 2 3 4 5	Encourages patients to express their thoughts and fears	0
6 Often uses terms not understood by patients	1 2 3 4 5	Uses terms easily understood by patients	0

	Ineffective		*Effective*	*Not appraised*
7	Makes no effort to meet family when indicated	1 2 3 4 5	Makes special efforts to meet family when indicated	0
8	Does not involve patients in management planning	1 2 3 4 5	Involves patients in management planning	0
9	Becomes agitated when dealing with emotional or difficult patients	1 2 3 4 5	Calm when dealing with emotional or difficult patients	0
10	Unable to explain patient problems without unduly alarming patients	1 2 3 4 5	Explains problems in a reassuring but truthful manner	0

Circle the number that most closely reflects the registrar's performance in that area.

Aspect B

History taking and interviewing skills

This aspect is concerned with the registrar's effectiveness in history taking and interviewing.

	Ineffective		Effective	Not appraised
1	Seldom takes time to put patient at ease	1 2 3 4 5	Interviews in a manner to put patient at ease	0
2	Does not demonstrate basic interviewing skills	1 2 3 4 5	Effectively uses basic interviewing skills	0
3	Has little control over the course of the interview	1 2 3 4 5	Conducts the interview in an orderly manner	0
4	Frequently asks the same question	1 2 3 4 5	Listens carefully	0
5	Interrupts or cuts patients short	1 2 3 4 5	Listens to patient's perception of problem	0
6	Takes inadequate or ritualistic histories	1 2 3 4 5	Elicits accurate and appropriate history	0
7	Interview too hurried or too drawn out	1 2 3 4 5	Interview length seems appropriate	0

	Ineffective							*Effective*	*Not appraised*
8	Misses opportunities to clarify information	1	2	3	4	5	Asks for clarification as necessary and explores appropriate leads		0
9	Fails to identify the patient's agenda	1	2	3	4	5	Uncovers the patient's motives for attendance		0
10	Does not consider the patient's understanding of his or her illness	1	2	3	4	5	Considers the patient's perception of his or her illness		0

Circle the number that most closely reflects the registrar's performance in that area.

Aspect C

Physical examination

This aspect is concerned with the registrar's effectiveness when physically examining patients.

	Ineffective						Effective	Not appraised
1	Fails to convey an impression of confidence	1	2	3	4	5	Handles patients in a reassuring manner	0
2	Fails to warn patients of the next step in examination	1	2	3	4	5	Informs patients of steps in examination as they proceed	0
3	Causes embarrassment to patients during examination	1	2	3	4	5	Is considerate during examination	0
4	Performs inadequate or unnecessary examinations	1	2	3	4	5	Examinations are accurate and appropriate	0
5	Tends to be disorganised when examining	1	2	3	4	5	Conducts systematic examinations	0
6	Is slow in examinations	1	2	3	4	5	Proceeds quickly and efficiently	0
7	Fails to recheck doubtful features	1	2	3	4	5	Rechecks doubtful, significant features	0

	Ineffective						*Effective*	*Not appraised*
8	Clumsy/ inadequate disorganised examinations for:						Deft and thorough examinations for:	
	head/neck	1	2	3	4	5	head/neck	0
	CVS	1	2	3	4	5	CVS	0
	RS	1	2	3	4	5	RS	0
	GI	1	2	3	4	5	GI	0
	GUS	1	2	3	4	5	GUS	0
	CNS	1	2	3	4	5	CNS	0
	LMS	1	2	3	4	5	LMS	0

Circle the number that most closely reflects the registrar's performance in that area.

Aspect D

Use of investigations

This aspect is concerned with the registrar's effectiveness when using laboratory and other facilities to gather and interpret results.

		Ineffective		Effective	Not appraised
1		Orders tests unrelated to identified problems	1 2 3 4 5	Discriminating in use of tests and other facilities	0
2		Has no clear rationale for ordering tests	1 2 3 4 5	Has clear rationale for tests ordered	0
3		Fails to integrate results into the overall clinical picture	1 2 3 4 5	Integrates results into the whole clinical scenario	0
4		Unaware of normal ranges of common tests	1 2 3 4 5	Aware of the normal range of common GP tests	0
5		Unaware of costs of tests	1 2 3 4 5	Aware of and considers costs of ordering tests	0
6		Unaware of patient's discomfort in proposed investigations	1 2 3 4 5	Considers patient discomfort and explains this appropriately	0

	Ineffective		*Effective*	*Not appraised*
7	Makes no attempt to discuss doubtful, significant, unusual results with colleagues	1 2 3 4 5	Discusses unusual findings with colleagues	0

Circle the number that most closely reflects the registrar's performance in that area.

Aspect E

Problem solving and clinical judgement

This aspect is concerned with the registrar's knowledge about health and disease, and his or her ability to assess a problem and develop a sound management plan.

	Ineffective		*Effective*	*Not appraised*
1	Difficulty in identifying problems accurately	1 2 3 4 5	Accurately identifies problems	0
2	Poor recall of factual information generally	1 2 3 4 5	Sound knowledge base	0
3	Cannot integrate factual knowledge in problem solving picture	1 2 3 4 5	Integrates factual knowledge in problem solving	0
4	Does not think of common conditions when appropriate	1 2 3 4 5	Considers common conditions to the appropriate degree	0
5	Has a poor idea of problem priorities	1 2 3 4 5	Prioritises problems maturely	0

	Ineffective		Effective	Not appraised
6	Unable to interpret unexpected findings and tends to ignore them	1 2 3 4 5	Responds to unexpected findings seeking to understand their significance	0
7	Leaves unusually loose ends in problem formulation	1 2 3 4 5	Takes all information into account to test alternative hypotheses	0
8	Frequently unable to determine the cause of common problems	1 2 3 4 5	Able to recognise the aetiology of common GP presentations	0
9	Shows little initiative in problem solving in practice	1 2 3 4 5	Shows inventiveness and skill in problem solving	0

Circle the number that most closely reflects the registrar's performance in that area.

Aspect F

Implementation of management plans

This aspect is concerned with the registrar's understanding and effectiveness in the provision of optimal patient care.

	Ineffective		Effective	Not appraised
1	Has little concept of and uses of PHCT	1 2 3 4 5	Integrates PHCT into normal daily practice	0
2	Has little concept of and rarely uses community resources	1 2 3 4 5	Integrates available community resources in his/her practice	0
3	Instructions are incomplete, inaccurate or disorganised	1 2 3 4 5	Instructions are comprehensive, logical and correct	0
4	Pays little attention to the side effects of drugs	1 2 3 4 5	Well aware of drug side effects and communicates relevant details	0
5	Ambiguous, hedging and contradictory in explanation to patients	1 2 3 4 5	Discusses findings and recommendations frankly and appropriately	0

	Ineffective							Effective	Not appraised
6	Does not instruct patients clearly and does not check understanding	1	2	3	4	5	Instructions are clear and checked	0
7	Misses opportunities to practise health education or prevention	1	2	3	4	5	Adept at integrating health education and preventative medicine into daily practice	0
8	Tends to use set routines or changes treatment with little attention to basic therapeutics	1	2	3	4	5	Flexible in treatment, modifying therapy and reassessing problems as appropriate	0

Circle the number that most closely reflects the registrar's performance in that area.

Curricular aims-related method

The A–Z objectives scale

This scale provides a series of aims across the spectrum of the curriculum. It does not purport to be all-inclusive. However, all the major elements of the curriculum are mentioned in one section or another, i.e. computers may be covered in many sections but if not, then the organisation section will pick that up. It is best used openly by both registrar and trainer.

A Introductory course
Aims
1 Buildings: – familiarise with own room and other clinical areas
– familiarise with alarms, keys
2 Equipment: – be able to access all the necessary equipment both personal and within the practice as a whole
3 Procedures: – familiar with note system, call system, appointment system
– aware of referral system, investigation system
– aware of how to access help (cover arrangements)
– aware of visit system
– aware of PHCT roles and availability
– aware of telephone system
4 Forms: – familiar with prescription and sickness certification forms
5 On call: – aware of issues of security, cover, necessary equipment and necessary contact numbers
6 Aware of relevant practice protocols (chaperones, disease management, video use, complaints, etc.)

---

7 Start personal administrative systems including educational strategies

B Audit/research

Aims

1 To be familiar with the principles and processes of audit
2 To be able to discuss the difference between audit and research
3 To perform a satisfactory audit
4 To develop a satisfactory attitude to audit/self-assessment

C Child health

Aims

1 To have a working knowledge of common children's illnesses
2 To be able to perform and understand the basis of child health screening and be eligible to enter the CHS list
3 To be able to examine children of all ages
4 To develop a personal and justifiable approach to referral of children
5 To be aware of the approaches to the care of chronically ill children
6 To feel comfortable managing children's problems (including parents)

D Chronic disease management

Aims

1 To understand the principles of chronic disease management
2 To understand the role of teamwork
3 To develop a personal and professional approach to the management of common chronic disease
4 To understand the role of referral

5 To understand the effects of chronic disease on patients/families/society
6 To understand the effects on the doctor of chronic disease management

E Common symptoms
Aims
1 To be able to manage common symptom presentations
2 To understand the concepts of symptom generation and presentation

F Complementary medicine
Aims
1 To be aware of the range of complementary therapies and their use
2 To develop an appropriate set of attitudes to complementary medicine
3 To know how to acquire skills in these areas if desired

G Consultation I
Aims
1 To develop an awareness of consultation dynamics
2 To explore ways of examining this process as a means to improving outcomes
3 To explore the range of interventions/behaviours available and ways of experimenting with these comfortably
4 To develop an awareness of the way the doctor's personality/feelings are affected by and can be used in the consultation

Consultation II
Aims
1 To establish goals for change
2 To develop strategies to achieve change

3 To implement and assess the effectiveness of these changes

4 To develop a long-term attitude to improving these skills

5 To be able to pass summative assessment video analysis and the MRCGP if desired

H Dermatology

Aims

1 To develop a diagnostic approach to rashes

2 To be able to recognise and to develop management plans for the common presentations (including referral)

I ENT

Aims

1 To be able to perform an ENT examination

2 To be able to recognise and manage the common presentations (including referral)

J Ethics

Aims

1 To be aware of the ethical principles at work in medicine

2 To develop an acceptable application of these principles

K Eyes

Aims

1 To be able to perform an ophthalmic examination (including lid eversion, use of fluorescein, colour perception and visual acuity)

2 To be able to recognise and manage the common presentations (including referral)

L Family planning
Aims
1 To be knowledgeable of the full range of family planning methods
2 To be trained to apply as many of these as felt appropriate
3 To be aware of the ethical issues in this field of medicine

M Gynaecology
Aims
1 To be able to perform a gynaecological examination (including use of various speculae and taking a smear and swabs
2 To be able to recognise and manage the common presentations (including referral)

N Infectious disease/immunisation
Aims
1 To be able to recognise and manage the range of infectious disease presentations
2 To know the theory and practice of immunisation. To be able to give all kinds of injections

O MRCGP
Aims
1 To be able to pass the MRCGP if desired

P Obstetrics
Aims
1 To know the theory and application of antenatal and postnatal care and to be able to perform the necessary procedures (including administrative)
2 To develop an appropriate attitude to and skill set for intrapartum care

Q Organisation

Aims

1 To feel personally organised on a:
   - patient-to-patient basis
   - day-to-day basis
   - week-to-week basis
   - long-term basis
2 To have an appreciation of management skills in this area
3 To identify personal areas of need and strategies to deal with these
4 To have an understanding of how organisations function, particularly those relevant to primary care
5 To have an understanding of the role of computers and IT in the health service and to be computer literate to an appropriate extent
6 To have an understanding of the relevant staff management issues
7 To have an understanding of the relevant financial management issues

R Personal and professional development

Aims

1 To develop an acceptable framework/system/attitude to continued professional and personal growth
2 To develop a sense of need in this area
3 To develop a sense of progress in this area
4 To be aware of the range of possibilities in this area
5 To be aware of the common problems in this area and strategies to deal with/prevent these

S Psychiatry

Aims

1 To understand the principles of brief psycho-therapy/counselling and similar activities within the consultation

2 To develop skills in counselling/brief psycho-therapy to an appropriate degree
3 To be able to recognise and manage common presentations (including referral) of psychiatric illness
4 To recognise the psychosocial aspects of many consultations
5 To understand the effect these problems can have on the doctor

T Rheumatology and orthopaedics
Aims
1 To be able to examine all joints
2 To be able to recognise and manage common presentations (including referral)
3 To develop special skills in this area if desired (joint aspiration/injection)

U Screening and prevention
Aims
1 To have an understanding of public health medicine and epidemiology
2 To understand the theory and practice of health promotion and screening
3 To be aware of the current screening programmes
4 To develop an acceptable attitudinal set in this area
5 To be able to demonstrate preventive activity in the consultation

V Substance abuse
Aims
1 To be aware of the common presentations of drug abuse
2 To have management skills in this area (including referral)
3 To develop an acceptable attitude in this area

W Surgical skills

Aims

1 To develop minor surgical skills as desired
2 To be aware of the necessary practice requirements for a minor surgery service
3 To be able to get on the minor surgery list if desired

X Teams

Aims

1 To know the requirements of a functional team
2 To acquire team building, leading and maintenance skills
3 To develop self-awareness in this area

Y Terminal care

Aims

1 To develop an appropriate attitude to death and dying
2 To acquire the necessary symptom management knowledge and skills
3 To develop an appreciation of the use of the PHCT in this area
4 To understand the patient and family perspectives of dying, death and grief
5 To understand the use of the various referral options in this area

Z Therapeutics I

Aims

1 To be aware of the full range of prescribing options
2 To know one's limitations in this area
3 To know how to access help in this area
4 To understand and demonstrate the principles of safe prescribing
5 To understand the resource implications
6 To develop evidence-based prescribing protocols for common conditions

Therapeutics II

Aims

1 To identify contentious issues in prescribing (i.e. costs, drug budgets, dispensing, drug companies, etc.)
2 To understand repeat prescribing systems
3 To develop a durable method of keeping up to date

List-based methods

The 'difficult' list

This is a short list produced by a group of registrars to highlight difficult presentations that seem to crop up early in the year:

► Termination requests
► Contraception in general
► Tired all the time
► Angry patients
► Critical patients
► The non-urgent 'extra'
► Patients 'demanding' a certain treatment (e.g. antibiotics)
► Depressed patients
► Headaches
► Admitting you are wrong/don't know what's wrong.

A survey of established GPs revealed the following list of common problems (from the UBC Residents Handbook):

► Achieving compliance (concordance)
► Diagnostic uncertainty
► Achieving appropriate follow-up
► Failure or absence of any treatment
► Inadequate resources
► Personal emotional reactions
► Time management
► Too many patients
► Staying up to date/training
► Knowing precise indications for interventions
► Waiting lists (investigations and hospitals)
► Access to and demand from non-medical services
► Patient expectations
► Sharing understanding with patients.

These lists encourage thought prior to the presentation of the problem and legitimise help-seeking behaviour. The lists could be endless of course!

Space for more!

Forms you should know

This list is intended as a guide to help you become aware of the range of paperwork that surrounds general practice.

▸ Collect an example of each of these forms.
▸ Try and find the latest *Pulse* Blue Book, which illustrates most of these forms nicely.
▸ Tick the ones you feel confident about.

Essentials

FP10 and variants (e.g. amounts/charges/ exemptions/limited list/DDAs)	......
Fmed3	......
Fmed4	......
Fmed5	......
Fmed6	......
RM7	......
Private sick notes	......
SC2	......
Private scripts	......
GMS4 (i.e. night visits/Reg. exam./ contraception/vaccs/minor ops, etc.)	......
Day-to-day practice paperwork (e.g. worksheets)	......
Investigation forms	......
Referral paperwork – general/physio/ chiropractic, etc.	......
Note-related paperwork	......

Related to pregnancy

GMS2	......
Mat B1	......
FW8	......
Newborn registration forms	......

Related to registration

GMS1   ......
GMS3 (temp services)   ......

Other administrative

Cremation certificates   ......
Target claim forms   ......
Insurance-related forms (reports/
    examinations/brief reports)   ......
Solicitor reports   ......
Seat belt exemptions   ......
DS1500 (special rules attendance allowance) ......
Disability and attendance allowance forms   ......
Overseas vaccination forms (cholera/
    yellow fever)   ......
HGV and taxi forms   ......
Occupational health forms   ......
Prescription exemption forms   ......
Claim for RTA attendance
    (Section 155 of 1972 Road Traffic Act)   ......
Abortion Act forms   ......
Wheelchair forms   ......
PACT and IPA forms   ......
DRO form (DP1)   ......

Other forms you should be aware of

PCG forms   ......
Annual reports   ......
Dispensing claim forms   ......

The ethics and law core curriculum

This is described in the *BMJ* **316**: 1624 (1998) and can act as a guide to covering ethical issues. It covers the following areas:

1 Informed consent
2 The clinical relationship (truth, trust and communication)
3 Confidentiality
4 Medical research
5 Human reproduction
6 The new genetics
7 Children
8 Mental disorders
9 Life, death, dying and killing
10 Vulnerabilities created by the duties of doctors
11 Resource allocation
12 Rights

A number of other useful references covering this area are mentioned in the articles listed in Chapter 10.

The 'need to know' list

The good practice of medicine is intertwined with the possession of good administrative skills. There are many administrative processes and systems at work in the practice – many of them do not involve you directly. The list below tries to provide a guide to those you should try and understand, in a priority order – often you will become aware as you are working but if in doubt *ask*.

Priority 1
► calling a patient
► initiating investigations
► referring patients
► writing a prescription
► writing in the notes or on computer
► claiming for contraception fees
► the repeat prescribing system
► temporary resident system
► minimum other 'essential' computer use
► other essential practice idiosyncratic systems

Priority 2
► visits system
► appointment system
► use of PHCT
► other potential consultation-related computer uses
► use of range of equipment in surgery
► dispensing rules (if appropriate)

Priority 3
► on-call systems/equipment
► knowledge of all computer use
► the financial systems at work
► other practice policies/systems
► audit systems
► complaints procedure
► staff management processes

Remember we have never had a registrar who asked too many questions!

NHSE basic computer skills list

Learning expectations

Health professionals should learn to:

1 organise electronic information (e.g. naming documents, setting up directories, moving files renaming files)
2 use a word processor package to generate simple documents
3 enter and manipulate data on a spreadsheet
4 search a simple database
5 undertake searches and access relevant sites on the web
6 retrieve and download documents from various sources and transfer data from one application to another
7 explain the reason for electronic networking and give examples of its use in the healthcare arena
8 send, receive and acknowledge e-mail and attachments
9 identify examples of the use of information technology as an effective tool in the delivery and management of healthcare
10 evaluate the effective use of information systems in the NHS. Discuss why different examples should be paper-based or electronic.

The following also need to be considered by some healthcare professionals:

11 set up a modem and internet connection
12 construct and deliver a computerised slide presentation
13 describe the data standards that exist for relevant operational systems, accessing networks and networked information.

CHAPTER 6

Tutorial planning: how do trainers plan tutorials?

It is always wise to look ahead but difficult to look farther than you can see

Churchill

Introduction

Many of the tools mentioned throughout this manual are designed to be used in a tutorial setting. So what is this chapter about? This section describes how trainers performed two tasks: first, how did they plan the format of the tutorial? and second, how did they find out if the tutorial 'worked'? The chapter finishes with an overview of tutorial planning. Trainers should ask themselves a critical question at this point: 'When do I learn best?'. The answer seems to lie in four main areas:

► when I need to, i.e. when I am aware of it and its relevance
► when I want to, i.e. when both the atmosphere and my attitude is suitable
► when I can, i.e. when the opportunity and the situation allow it
► when it works, i.e. I see its value.

Trainers need to apply the practicalities of these points. Tutorials need to be relevant (sometimes difficult because they can be perceived as detached from the clinical core of the work) and jointly agreed. The trainer and registrar must create a suitable environment and feel positive about the potential for learning. The time should be protected, valued and 'seized'. *Carpe diem* (seize the day) encapsulates the concept that learning opportunities can be fleeting moments and should be grasped firmly as they arise – again difficult to achieve in the protected time tutorial. Trainers need to look for these moments from day to day and patient to patient. Finally trainers need to create the environment where the value of new learning can be tested and proved. These points are the challenge to trainers as they plan the tutorial programme.

Tutorial structure

The trainer's approach

Many trainers have evolved their own tutorial assessment scales. An analysis of these reveals a number of commonalities:

1 a subject area was identified jointly
2 aims and objectives in this area were jointly negotiated
3 the method to tackle these aims was negotiated with enjoyment high on the agenda
4 the timing, setting and facilitator were agreed
5 the process occurred
6 the registrar was asked for feedback in six areas:
   – relevance
   – whether aims were achieved, and what was learnt
   – what worked well?
   – what could have been better?
   – enjoyment
   – need for follow-up work
7 the feedback was jointly reviewed.

The forms varied in their design: some were purely feedback and others combined this with a recording function and acted as a training log. The latter seems to have practical advantages. The Appendix to Chapter 5 contains a form combining these elements.

The assessor's approach

Many regions now actively try to assess trainers' teaching skills. The most common approach is the video assessment of a tutorial and in some areas this could soon be a compulsory component of reapproval for training.

Does the process used for this assessment help us plan the tutorial – maybe! It will *definitely* help trainers produce a reasonable video of the tutorial and this *may* improve the learning process.

Two models of the tutorial process are discussed by Ruscoe (1994) describing a task and a process analysis. These are shown in Boxes 6.1 and 6.2.

Box 6.1: Task-orientated model of tutorial

1 Learner need jointly identified
2 Learning need discussed
3 Learning need agreed
4 Teaching strategy proposed
5 Teaching strategy agreed
6 Teaching strategy implemented
7 Future needs identified
8 Future needs discussed
9 Future needs agreed

> **Box 6.2: Process model of tutorial**
>
> 1 Introduction
> 2 Baggage check
> 3 Exploration
> 4 Discovery
> 5 Planning
> 6 Evaluation

The major concept these models add to the trainer-based approach is the idea of 'baggage checking'. This is the tutorial equivalent of housekeeping. It is useful to highlight the need to resolve any outstanding personal, clinical or educational demands that would impede the learning process *before* you start. The process model also highlights the issue of planning and emphasises that the tutorial is part of a process and should not be seen in isolation.

The qualitative aspects of teaching also come under scrutiny by the assessors. These can be looked at under a number of headings:

1 Structural – does the training happen in a good environment in protected time?
2 Process – is the process learner-centred, flexible, sensitive and stimulating?
3 Outcomes – are these sought and considered maturely?

The whole process should occur in the context of an appropriate trainer/registrar relationship. The Appendix to Chapter 5 contains an assessment form combining these points.

Style

All trainers teach in style – of course they do. But *what* style? Heron (1986) produced a description of different facilitation styles that could be adopted by trainers as they performed various tasks. This model challenges the trainer to assess whether they use the appropriate style consistently.

He describes three modes of facilitation each usable in six dimensions producing the grid shown in Table 6.1.

Table 6.1: Facilitation

Dimensions	Modes		
	Hierarchical	Cooperative	Autonomous
Planning			
Setting objectives and assessments	Trainer plans but does not really negotiate	Trainer negotiates and coordinates	Trainer delegates
Meaning			
Making sense of and understanding the task and process of learning	Trainer inputs theory, interprets and assesses	Trainer asks neutral questions (What is happening now?), uses descriptive feedback and negotiates assessment	Trainer uses reflection Group self-assesses and self-analyses Trainer may even delegate this role
Confronting			
Raising awareness about blocks in learning enabling self-confrontation	Trainer interprets and may even describe block	Trainer describes events and asks for views on avoidance	Trainer provides environment that is safe
Feeling			
Identify negative emotional processes, interrupt them and alter them.	Trainer decides how feelings are managed and thinks for the group.	Trainer works with the group to develop ways to cope with feelings	Trainer gives space to manage feelings
Achieving a balance of emotions	Trainer gives permission for catharsis		

Table 6.1: continued

Dimensions	Modes		
	Hierarchical	Cooperative	Autonomous
Structuring			
Giving form to the learning process	Trainer takes over the design and supervision	Trainer cooperates to let rules emerge using counselling skills	Trainer delegates design
Valuing			
Creating climate of respect	Trainer uses actions and commitment, i.e. charisma Trainer has positive regard for others	Trainer collaborates to allow self-respect and favourable climate to emerge	Trainer lets the group determine its own climate Makes self-disclosures on values

Some trainers adopt a very hierarchical approach to structuring, a cooperative approach to valuing and an autonomous one to confronting. The model challenges trainers to consider the appropriate style for each situation.

Quirk (1994) describes four types of teaching style:

▶ Assertive-style teaching: extrovert and tends to direct the process by leading from the front.

▶ Suggestive-style teaching: tends to offer ideas and thoughts readily.

▶ Collaborative-style teaching: identifies and legitimises the learner's difficulties.

▶ Facilitative-style teaching: encourages the learner to discover the way forward using and developing their own skills.

The model can be interpreted to imply that all good trainers should always use a facilitative style. Even if it is accepted as an ideal, this style will be ineffective and inappropriate in some situations. The underconfident registrar may need the trainer to give an answer before feeling able to offer his or her own; many registrars will face situations where they can see no options and require prompting with a range of suggestions. In these situations it may be ideal to encourage the registrar to develop his or her confidence or research the problem – but trainers have to operate in the real world where confidence is not built up overnight and patients can't wait 30 minutes while the registrar looks something up. The models can help trainers become more aware of the style options and increase their repertoire of options.

Theory

These are my principles and if you don't like them, I have others

Anon

Role modelling/coaching	Johari's window	Competency model
Educational triangle	Field dependence	Hemispheric dominance

When trainers were asked 'Is educational theory useful?' the most common response was 'No!'. On the basis of 'no pain, no gain', *some* trainers found *some* of the theory useful. This section is a brief description of which bits, where and how. Give it a read and who knows?

Role modelling, apprenticeship and coaching

Even within the English-speaking Western World, training systems for primary care physicians are incredibly variable. The common themes seem to be role modelling, apprenticeship and coaching. The most influential, stimulating and exciting training programmes will ultimately rise or fall depending on the individuals that learners can role model themselves upon.

Descriptions of excellent learning environments stress the presence of good role models. Most doctors have little problem naming at least one influential role model in their own education. These people have often demonstrated mastery in a particular area. They have usually combined this with *caritas* and the feeling of contentment derived from a job well done. Each learner models themselves on a variety of individuals to a variable degree and much of this learning is at the unconscious level for both the learner and the role model. The trainer can attempt to influence this process in a number of ways:

▶ by raising awareness in the learner and trainers that this process is at work to try and move the experience into the conscious sphere
▶ highlighting the positive features of a particular role model
▶ highlighting the negative features of a particular role model to avoid poor role modelling and attempt to create counterpoint features for modelling
▶ to consciously expose the learner to role models who demonstrate attributes the learner (and/or trainer) perceives as their own educational needs.

These observations and the attributes of the ideal primary care physician (*see* Table 3.1) represent a challenge to trainers and to those who approve training practices. While it may be possible to increase registrars' awareness of these desirable qualities, the apprenticeship model illustrates that the qualities actually observed and experienced will be more influential.

The stages of apprenticeship offer some insights for the training practice:

I   Observation: apprentices observe – warts and all! They *see* things go well and not so well.

II   Modelling: without any other input the apprentice starts to model his or her behaviour on what they observe. At this stage he or she cannot reliably identify which behaviours are most desirable. (Think of how young children often demonstrate their parents' most irritating habits!)

III   Articulation: the trainer describes how to perform the skill. The apprentice questions and demonstrates understanding at the verbal level.

IV   Demonstration: the trainer demonstrates the process to the apprentice; the apprentice demonstrates the process, with support and protection from the trainer.

V   Withdrawal: the trainer slowly withdraws under control.

VI   Independence: the apprentice has acquired independent skill.

VII   Generalising: the trainer encourages the apprentice to analyse new skills, develop principles and use these to solve new problems.

VIII   Coaching: the trainer encourages the accomplished apprentice to identify areas and techniques for possible refinement.

(Coaching is the process of enhancing the performance and learning ability of others, using motivation, effective questioning, feedback and personality style awareness techniques.)

This process describes how registrars learn many new skills. Often the learning has an implicit element and trainers are using these concepts subconsciously (unconscious competence; *see* next section). An explicit awareness can be helpful if problem situations arise (poor role modelling) or a particular problem emerges (attach the anxious registrar to the most relaxed partner?).

Johari's window

This is a pictorial model that aims to aid understanding of where change might occur. It is shown in Figure 6.1.

The theory states that you learn more as you open up the arena. You do this by reducing the blind spot and the hidden agenda. As the axes move, you necessarily reduce the closed area too. So what does this mean in practical terms? This tool is useful to convey your philosophy of training to the 'theorist-type' registrar, particularly if you feel there is an element of reticence in giving and receiving feedback. In practical terms, it encourages positive attitudes to self-disclosure and feedback.

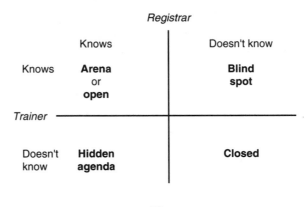

Figure 6.1: Johari's window.

Competency model

This is a model to describe the process of learning a new skill. It is shown in Figure 6.2.

The theory holds that we move from unconscious incompetence to unconscious competence. It is helpful in a number of ways:

▶ it reminds registrars that new skills are just over the horizon

► it reminds registrars that they have unconsciously competent skills already

► it highlights that the process of learning includes a period of conscious incompetence, i.e. they are going to feel uncomfortable and if they don't something is wrong!

► it reminds trainers that to teach something it helps to be consciously competent to some degree (and also that they too have unconscious incompetences!).

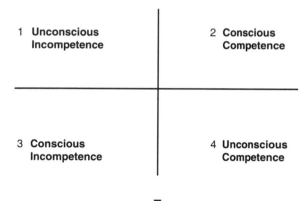

Figure 6.2: The competency model.

Educational triangle

Figures 6.3 and 6.4 show the educational triangle in two forms. The first is the conventional model and the second emphasises the processes involved. Many registrars come into general practice with years of didactic, ritually humiliating educational experience. Some of the approaches GP trainers use are completely novel to them. They have acquired all sorts of educational myths, i.e. 'all assessment is summative and I must produce the right answers' or 'admitting you don't know is a sign of weakness'. It helps to give them insight to the formative nature of the process. This can be done simply with a diagram (for the visual learner), as a discussion (perhaps for the reflector) or you can make a series of cards and play with them on the floor (for the activist). It is helpful to point out that each element of the process-type educational triangle has its own internal triangle also – even make a set of smaller cards to illustrate the point.

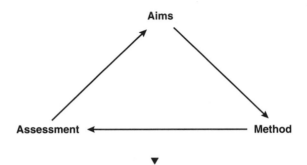

Figure 6.3: The conventional educational cycle.

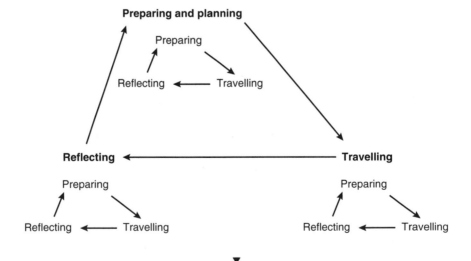

Figure 6.4: The process educational cycle.

The cycle is more accurately described as a spiral and this concept helps to reinforce that we all get second, third, fourth and perhaps limitless opportunities to learn as problems re-present. This gives us the dual opportunities of reinforcing past learning and looking for more insights in the light of that learning. This type of exercise can significantly alter a registrar's attitude to the learning process.

Field dependence model

This is a model of learning styles developed by Riding and Cheema (1991). It contains a number of concepts, but the field dependency idea can have practical value. The characteristics of field-dependent/independent types are shown in Box 6.3.

Box 6.3: Characteristics of field-dependent/ independent learners

Field-dependent learners	Field-independent learners
Relate to peers well	Require little interaction with peers
Use external frames of reference	Use internal frame of reference
Need external reinforcement	Intrinsic reinforcement
Need structured work	Structure own learning needs
Good interpersonal skills	Need help in developing social skills
Need help problem solving	Good at problem solving

If the trainer can recognise their registrar's field dependency then it can be used to design appropriate facilitation methods. It is also useful for trainers to identify their own field dependency preferences (Box 6.4).

Box 6.4: Characteristics of field-dependent/ independent teachers

Field-dependent teachers	**Field-independent teachers**
Prefer interaction with learners	Prefer formal approaches
Are reluctant to express criticism	Emphasise their own standards
Are concerned with a positive atmosphere	Focus on content rather than attitudes or ambience

---

Hemispheric dominance theory

This theory holds that one side of our brain has a controlling dominance over some aspects of our thinking and behaviour. In *The Hemispheric Mode Indicator: right and left brain approaches to learning* (Barrington 1985) a technique is described to identify an individual's bias. Many feel this can be assessed just as readily by observation:

▸ Right dominant: creative, musical, rhythmical, intuitive, spontaneous.
▸ Left dominant: logical, organised, rational, controlled, deductive.

Teaching methods can then be tailored to fit the preferred instructional mode of the registrar. This concept is illustrated further in the Appendix to Chapter 5.

Feedback

We must remember to talk about goodness every day

Socrates

Most trainers find this a difficult area. This is probably related to our past humiliations at the hands of previous teachers and our enduring fear of failure. It is very difficult to give feedback if you still harbour these feelings. Successful feedback is given in an atmosphere where it is accepted as an essential and positive ingredient of the learning process. So basically you must give *and receive* it regularly, openly, honestly, positively *and* negatively. Box 6.5 shows the principles that should be used.

Box 6.5: Principles for feedback

- Owned (i.e. use of 'I' not 'we') NOT implied
- Planned NOT impulsive
- Honest NOT collusive
- Valid NOT irrelevant (i.e. apply to a shared agenda)
- Concerned NOT destructive
- Specific NOT vague
- Behaviour NOT the person
- Observation NOT inference
- Sooner NOT later
- Descriptive NOT judgemental
- Sharing ideas NOT giving advice
- Exploring alternatives NOT providing answers
- Good NOT only bad (i.e. balanced and reinforcing good learning)

The trainer needs courage, understanding, self-respect and skills as well as a respect for the registrar. The focus should be on behaviour that is amenable to change and the feedback should be prescribed in a manner analogous to drug prescribing, that is:

► correctly timed
► in the right dose (not too little or too much)
► with clarity and accuracy
► when the correct indication exists, i.e. the feedback will work
► with the registrar's concordance
► with explicit conditions for follow-up for the registrar's benefit (i.e. not the trainer's).

The 'feedback sandwich' is a practical reminder of the need to provide feedback with protection, particularly if you have an underconfident registrar. This simply implies you wrap the constructive criticism in two layers of positive comment. A lot of feedback is simple and straightforward, but the trainer needs to be sensitive to the feelings it can produce in the registrar before the feedback session is closed.

If this is an obvious problem for a registrar the following techniques can be tried:

► a tutorial where trainer/registrar describe the best/ worst feedback they have ever had
► a tutorial where the trainer and registrar role play a feedback scenario.

Trainers should always remember that a quick 'That's right! Well done' reinforces learning very effectively. Similarly negative feedback should be given without unnecessary repetition.

Specific teaching tools

Questions and answers

As long as the answer is right, who cares if the question is wrong?

Jung

Any parent will testify to the truth that asking questions is easier than answering them! One of the key skills in developing a registrar's self-directed learning approach is the use of appropriate questions. In the training environment, questions are not answered – they are questioned! Four types of question can be used:

1 Direct questions: a question seeking an answer or sequence of answers.
2 Probing questions:
   – with cues
   – with elaboration
   – with explanation
   – to provoke knowledge seeking
   – to involve others (perhaps in a group).
3 High order questions, i.e. broadening the area, seeking justifications. These are questions that provoke thought, bring out principles or require problem solving skills.
4 Divergent questions, i.e. hypotheses or alternatives-seeking questions that open awareness, often have no 'right' answer and encourage creative thinking.

Registrars can find these approaches frustrating if they are new to this kind of teaching. It can help if trainers make the reasons for this style explicit. It can be very rewarding when registrars produce their own solutions with a smile and the trainer hadn't even thought of one!

Teaching clinical skills

Teaching clinical examination and procedures

The following sequence has been suggested as a guide to use when teaching clinical skills in the clinical setting:

1 Set the environment.
2 Introduce and inform everyone.
3 Work out and describe the sequence of actions that are required.
4 Demonstrate the process as you would normally perform it.
5 Use imagery/models to illustrate the process.
6 Check the registrar's understanding of the process.
7 The registrar performs the process under supervision.
8 Focus sensory awareness on key elements (i.e. close eyes).
9 Build confidence with feedback and practice.
10 Use linking:
   - facts to feelings
   - visual to other sensory inputs
   - clinical history to examination findings.
11 Increase responsibility (registrar does it alone).
12 Check on progress at agreed time interval.

Although the points seem obvious, it does challenge the trainer to define the skills required and to develop a bank of teaching strategies and linkage techniques for this process. It can be an interesting exercise to take a commonly taught procedure (perhaps proctoscopy or ingrowing toenail (IGTN) surgery) and work it through these stages. Most trainers will find a number of aspects they had assumed (i.e. unconscious competence) the registrar was skilled in. These assumptions may, or may not, be correct and are usefully highlighted.

Teaching GP clinical strategies

Many registrars have developed a hospital-based approach to diagnosis and examination. Most learn to adapt this approach rapidly. The family medicine department at the University of British Columbia, Vancouver, raises this process to a conscious level by working through common presentations using a number of set questions. The form used is reproduced in the Appendix to Chapter 5. The process can be useful in two areas. First, to help the registrar who is having difficulty adapting to the primary care environment, and second, to look at a particular presentation that a registrar may be struggling with. Trainers need to consider the potential problem of giving the message that there is always a single set of 'right' questions for a particular presentation but, with this proviso, the method could be helpful.

The micro-lesson 'CATCH – ing' the learning opportunity

This phrase was coined by one trainer and coincides with a concept developed from Irby (1992) by Dr Bob Woollard in the family medicine department at UBC, Vancouver. Much of our 1:1 teaching involves short interactions with the registrar between consultations or actually with patients present. Five 'microskills' for the teacher can be developed to act as a guide to maximise the learning potential in this situation.

- ► **Commitment:** the trainer should ask the learner for a commitment to the problem (i.e. diagnosis, reason for attendance, problem definition). This involves clarification of the learner's knowledge base in relation to presentation and management issues.
- ► **Analysis:** the trainer should now ask for a demonstration of the reasoning behind the assessment. This

allows the learner's problem-solving skills to be demonstrated.

▶ **T**eaching: the trainer can now assess the need for new knowledge and help with problem solving. This is the time to bring out the principles or concepts that apply in the situation, i.e. some teaching.

▶ **C**ompliments: the power of positive feedback can never be underestimated. The trainer should say specifically what was done well and what effect this has had. Opportunities for reinforcement of good practice should never be missed.

▶ **H**owlers: obvious mistakes, omissions, misunderstandings should highlight learning needs and these should be appropriately fed back.

Problems of 1:1 teaching (*see* Chapter 9)

Table 6.2 describes some of the potential problem factors in the 1:1 teaching relationship. Generally the main problem behaviours are:

▶ trainer talking too much
▶ trainer telling the registrar how to do it or even trying to tell them everything
▶ trainer adopting a passive role and neglecting the stimulus role
▶ trainer avoiding areas they are uncomfortable with
▶ trainer using avoidance behaviour when uncomfortable (instead of feedback)
▶ trainer making quick judgements
▶ trainer interrogating
▶ trainer not listening
▶ trainer gives only negative feedback
▶ trainer failing to see the tutorial as part of a larger process.

The poem by RD Laing illustrates some of these areas (even if you do have to read it twice!)

A Knot by RD Laing

There is something I don't know
That I am supposed to know
I don't know what it is I don't know
And yet am supposed to know
I feel I look stupid
If I seem both not to know it
And not know what it is I don't know
Therefore I pretend I know it
This is nerve wracking
Since I don't know what I must pretend to know
Therefore I pretend to know everything
I feel you know what I am supposed to know
But you can't tell me what it is
Because you don't know that I don't know what it is
You may know what I don't know
But not that I don't know it
And I can't tell you
So you will have to tell me everything!

The point about listening bears some examination. Brown and Atkins (1988) describe five types of listening.

- ► *skim listening* – most is skimming past you as you think of something else
- ► *search listening* – you are scanning for a particular point
- ► *survey listening* – taking an overview without the detail (when did you last listen to the story of someone's holiday?)
- ► *study listening* – paying attention to all the words said and what they convey
- ► *deep study listening* – looking for meaning in the words and non-verbal communication and trying to understand the reasons and feelings behind them.

Trainers need to adopt the same listening skills they use in the consultation in their teaching environment.

Table 6.2: Factors that impair learning

Registrar	Trainer	Registrar/Trainer
Poor preparation	Too technical	Poor rapport
Poor confidence	Too didactic	Collusive
Anxiety	Too talkative	Allow parent/child
Introversion	Too impressive	relationship
	Too self-centred	
	Too judgemental	
	Too inattentive	

Other points to note

Communication

It has been said that input into the human brain occurs
in the following proportions:

- sight   70%, a major input and major distraction
- sound   20%
- touch   5%
- taste/smell 5%.

The second commonly quoted 'fact' is that 60% of communication is at the non-verbal level. So demonstration,
use of visual-based material and non-verbal communication skills are vitally important in teaching. Messages
can be reinforced by combining visual, auditory, sensual
and affective inputs. This principle of 'linkage' seems to
increase the likelihood of retention of learning. The ability
of the brain to store and retrieve information is increased
if the learning is 'linked' to almost any other input: the
more links the better (to a degree), i.e. try and link learning to patients, places, times, feelings, diseases, sounds,
sights, smells, tastes, etc. And using the learner's VAK
preferences may improve the efficiency of the process. If
nothing else it should make the learning process varied
and fun.

Key phrases

These five phrases can act as a simple aide-mémoire in tutorials. Trainers should encourage the registrar to move from:

- the unknown to the known
- the concrete to the abstract
- the whole to the parts
- the simple to the complex
- the general to the specific.

Problem-solving styles

One of the core skills of general practice is the ability to problem solve efficiently. How can trainers teach this? A clue may lie in the individuals problem solving style. Cox and Ewan (1988) described three styles, described below.

Pattern recognition

Much of our clinical training and experience results in an internalised data bank of clinical patterns. This recognition system seems to be active in the first few minutes of a consultation. If a pattern is not recognised within this time then it probably won't be at all. Pattern recognition requires knowledge and experience, but the trainer can try and imprint patterns on the registrar by highlighting them when seen and raising awareness of the pattern recognition system. One area where this works particularly well is in the diagnosis of rashes. However, the obvious visual input of a rash can provoke a premature pattern recognition response, i.e. I should know that because I can see it. In this situation the trainer can encourage the registrar to adopt a structured history and diagnosis technique, and to suspend premature 'diagnostic panic'. Then as more data is acquired a diagnostic pattern becomes apparent.

Diagnosis-directed search

If no pattern is discernible then the doctor initiates a search process. The initial symptoms and signs are analysed to produce a number of possible diagnoses (usually less than four or five). The internalised predictive values of these symptoms and signs are used to deduce the most likely diagnoses. Each diagnosis is then tested against the data until the probability diagnosis emerges. This testing is done in one of two ways: by *accumulating* and interpreting masses of data until the balance is tipped in favour of one diagnosis or by collecting a subset of data that possesses *discriminating* qualities that allow the diagnosis to emerge. The latter process tends to be more efficient. This is the hypothetical–deductive approach used in many consultations. It requires a knowledge base, experience (which can also mislead) and ideally an idea of the predictive values of symptoms and signs (which are often not available in a useful format). Trainers can facilitate this process by providing experience, highlighting knowledge deficits and encouraging a critical approach to the acquisition of new knowledge. New knowledge should have a discriminating quality. It is perhaps here that evidence-based medicine may help in the future.

Systematic enquiry

Many trainers will remember be taught the 'systems enquiry' element of history taking. Many will have asked a patient presenting with osteoarthritis of the knee if they had haemoptysis. Thankfully many medical schools have realised that this is probably not a good way to learn or practise. However, *systematic scanning* is performed by doctors regularly. When a diagnosis is elusive it can prove useful to scan for possible associated symptoms or signs that can complete the picture, i.e. with an unusual back pain, enquiry about eye symptoms may elicit the history of iritis and point towards a seronegative arthritis. Most doctors develop a series of scanning questions. They often start in a selected pattern (i.e. enquiry about eye, skin and bowel symptoms with arthritis) and can include opening 'screening'-type enquiry (i.e. anything wrong with your chest?) before going in a bit deeper if indicated (any cough?, any blood?, etc.). Raising awareness of this process can help registrars to make better use of the battery of questions available to them.

All three of these problem-solving styles are required in general practice. The art is to use the most efficient and effective style on the day. An awareness of the styles can help both registrars and trainers to try and achieve this.

Planning the tutorial – a skeleton guide

This section aims to summarise the tutorial planning process combining the methods described.

Table 6.3: Tutorial planning structure

Task		Potential methods
Find a learning area:	knowledge	Confidence rating scales/inventories
		MCQ or PEP tests
		Review of experience/qualifications
		RCA/Feedback from staff, patients, doctors
		Note, script, referral reviews
	skills	Observation and discussion (direct, video, etc.)
		Skills lists
		Specific areas (minor surgery, child health surveillance, contraception, examination techniques, etc.)
		Management (observation, feedback, experience, etc.)
	self-awareness	Observation, discussion and feedback

Table 6.3: Continued

Task	Potential methods
Find a learning area: statutory	Audit, trainer's report
other methods	Registrar wish list
	Specific lists (need to know, difficult list, ethics list, A–Z list, etc.)
	Personal construct analysis
	Review of reflective diary
	Review of problems raised by registrar (problem-based learning)
Jointly agree on learning needs	Jointly agree on aims
	Discussion and record on a tutorial planning document
	Assess learning style/personality
	Learning style questionnaire
	Self-directed learners rating scale (SDLRS)
	Myers–Briggs type indicator
	Field dominance, hemispheric dominance, VAK preference
	Assertiveness
	Thinking style
	Discussion
Assess motivation and skill level	Motivation scale, motivation cycles
	Observation and discussion
	Skill/will matrix
Jointly agree methods	Patient-based:
	▶ random or virtual case analysis
	▶ video mapping/SETGO/ Pendleton's rules/exam systems/ other lists/open observation/ models
	▶ joint surgeries
	▶ role playing

Table 6.3: Continued

Task	Potential methods
Jointly agree methods	Other methods: pictures/ pre-recorded videos/ written material (guidelines, articles, questionnaires, CASE booklets, prompt cards, etc.)/models/scripts or referral/reviews/juggling/'tips and tricks', etc.
Preparation and planning	Written on a planning form. May include reading (references, tutorial planning guides), 'thinking time', filling in questionnaires, collecting cases, using the internet, etc.
The tutorial event	Protected time and a suitable environment
	Appropriate resources
	'Baggage check', i.e. both registrar and trainer are ready to go
	The process with the trainer demonstrating:

- active listening
- appropriate questioning skills
- appropriate feedback skills
- use of a variety of educational tools
- the encouragement of self-awareness
- the development of problem solving skills
- appropriate information giving behaviour
- a sense of direction and position (i.e. not straying inappropriately off course)
- an awareness of any appropriate emotional elements
- enthusiasm and interest

Table 6.3: Continued

Task	Potential methods
Closing the tutorial	Reviewing aims, developing new aims
	Considering follow up sessions
	Ensuring final baggage check, i.e. are there any loose ends?
	Arranging for feedback – for both parties
	Use of tutorial record form

This scheme can produce the same feelings in a trainer as lists of the components of a primary care consultation expected to last 10 minutes can in the new registrar. When looked at as a whole, the structure simply raises to the conscious level the processes most trainers are already using to some degree. By doing this it opens up the possibility of reviewing the process and possibly improving it.

Summary comments

If you fail to plan, you are planning to fail

Anon

The art of facilitating the learning process involves juggling a number of variables. Registrars have different learning styles, they think using different cognitive styles, use different problem-solving styles and they have different preferences for learning environments (instructional preferences). Trainers have their own teaching styles and a toolbox of strategies to employ. Dovetailing these variables is the challenge.

Tutorial planning can make a huge difference to the quality of the training year. It is said there are only two real commodities in this world – time and space – and there isn't much of either! Trainers need to plan their time so they can plan their tutorials and this section may make that process a little easier.

Appendix to Chapter 6

The trainer's tutorial assessment form

This form combines the elements of at least 15 individual forms in current use. It aims to serve a number of functions:

► to act as record of the learning experience/tutorial
► to act as a planning aid
► to encourage feedback from the registrar and facilitator.

A Subject area

B Aims/objectives
1
2
3

C Date of activity and methods employed

D Registrar's comments
Please mark the scales as appropriate:

                    very enjoyable   not very enjoyable

Enjoyment   _____

Relevance   _____

Use of method _____

Please comment on: 1 Were our objectives reached?
                   2 Has this session raised new
                     objectives? (with description)
                   3 Any other comments at all?

Circle the words that describe how you feel about this tutorial:

Interested	Bored	Informative	Verbose
Motivated	Daunted	Useless	Disinterested
Relevant	Unnecessary		

E Facilitator name
   Facilitator comments: particularly on areas for development and comments relevant to this registrar.

Please return this form to the registrar
(The registrar must arrange for the trainer to receive a photocopy.)

Thank you

The assessor's tutorial assessment form

This is an amalgamation of at least three forms currently available for assessing tutorials. Generally they are applied after observing a tutorial (sitting in, video or role play). They have been used in trainers' workshops to look at tutorial skills.

TUTORIAL ASSESSMENT FORM

Competence   Exemplary 5 4 3 2 1   Poor   Comment

1 Preparation

2 Environment

3 Communication
(and baggage check)

4 Relationship

5 Learner-centred
► assessing needs
► setting aims
► choosing method

6 Appropriate structure
► time
► method
► develops registrar's
self-awareness
► develops registrar's
critical thinking

7 Flexibility

Competence	Exemplary	5 4 3 2 1	Poor	Comment

8 Evaluation
▶ by registrar
▶ by trainer

9 Future planning

Hemispheric dominance model

An appreciation of the registrar's and trainer's hemispheric dominance can provide some insights that could improve the learning process.

The table below can be used to inform the trainer.

Left dominant	Right dominant
Likes language, numbers, symbols	Likes pictures/images
Verbally expressive	Demonstrative
Controlled/systematic	Open-minded/random
Analytical	Creative
Prefers talking/writing	Prefers private studying
Looks for cause and effect	Experiential
Controls feelings	Free with feelings
Overskills himself/herself	Tends to underskill themselves
Reads first	Does first
Sense of time	Intuitive (often late!)
Objective	Subjective

Butler and Hermann (in Barrington 1985) added a further 'upper and lower' dimension to this model postulating a different role for the lower and upper cerebral hemispheres. This allowed the development of four learning styles that are described opposite.

Upper left **ABSTRACT SEQUENTIAL**	Upper right **ABSTRACT RANDOM**
Parts processed better than wholes. Orderly, sequential, analytical, systematic approaches. Wants schedules and precise instruction. Prefers to work independently with a rational and intellectual approach.	Sees the whole better than the parts. Prefers abstract concepts, patterns and creative approaches. Uses non-linear, intuitive and spontaneous styles. Works independently and likes to see the whole picture.
Lower left **CONCRETE SEQUENTIAL**	Lower right **CONCRETE RANDOM**
Steady, reliable, predictable and organised. Prefers words to shapes or concepts. Likes detail and follows instruction. Prefers to work with others. Needs encouragement. Dislikes surprises. Good listener. Likes defined problems.	Lives in the world of feelings, music, movement and relationships. Relies on doing and feeling. Sensitive to others' feelings and meanings. Restless if not doing. Likes fun. Likes others. Needs to dream, create and be challenged.

Eric Jensen (1994) describes the parallels between child and adult learning in his book *Superteaching* and encourages more 'fun and play' with adults. He suggests the following ideal circumstances to maximise learning:

► lots of play (i.e. games, tricks, activities)
► humour (encouraging laughter)
► imagination (abstract props, interpretation)
► positive support (encouragement, reinforcement, praise)
► relaxation (more play, social activities)
► physical activity (walks, games, etc.)
► use of music and singing (tapes, videos)

- a rich environment – visually and physically (resources, inspiration, motivation)
- a good peer group.

GP clinical strategies form

This form is a series of questions to work through. The aim is to investigate the techniques that GPs use to manage presentations, particularly in relation to the time restraints at work in primary care.

- What is the problem/presentation?
- What is the worst case scenario?
- What are the essential questions?
- What are the 'red flags'?
- What investigations are indicated?
- What aspects of the patients agenda might be relevant?
- Are there any health education aspects of relevance?
- Does the trainer know of any 'pearls of wisdom' on this subject?

Useful presentations to consider include:

- TATT
- URTIs
- rashes
- joint pains
- headaches
- sleep problems
- chest pains
- SOB, etc.

CHAPTER 7

Management and change: how do trainers cover practice management issues and the concepts of management of change?

We trained hard, but it seemed that every time we were beginning to form up into new teams we would be reorganised. I was to learn later in life that we tend to meet any new situation by reorganising and a wonderful method it can be for creating the illusion of progress while producing confusion, inefficiency and demoralisation

Petronius, Roman General AD 66

Introduction

A survey of newly vocationally trained GPs identified practice and staff management as areas of perceived deficiency in their training. This is partly explained by Laing's poem *The Knot* (*see* Chapter 6). Many registrars 'Don't know what they are supposed to know' and only find out in practice. However, the trainer does have a duty to raise awareness of this blindspot. This section describes the methods trainers use to try and achieve this aim.

The 'why' of management

A tutorial based on this question can open up awareness. The following areas could be raised for discussion. Is the function of managing to:

- ▶ Educate people?
- ▶ Focus effort?
- ▶ Get the job done?
- ▶ Direct people because there only seems to be one solution?
- ▶ Be safe?
- ▶ Be efficient?
- ▶ Prevent problems?
- ▶ Get revenge?
- ▶ Prevent mistakes?
- ▶ Make things easier?
- ▶ Reward?
- ▶ Have control?

One trainer suggested contrasting a 'well-managed' organisation with a 'badly managed' one to bring out these points. The principles of total quality management (a Japanese industrial tool where everyone is seen as a valuable contributor to a business at every level) can also be discussed.

The 'how' of management

Personal management skills	Action planning	GROW, SMART and FRAME
Navigation theory	POSSEER	Cognitive therapy
Logical levels	SWOT	Others

Personal management

Anyone who has had more than one child will realise people seem to be fundamentally different from an early age. While it may be optimistic to expect dramatic changes in an individual's behaviour it is possible to offer practical tips.

Practical tips

An interesting distinction exists between the words important and urgent. Many of us spend a lot of time doing 'urgent' things. Urgency is usually defined by the needs of others, important things relate to our own needs. On occasions we need to reflect on whether the urgent task we are doing is more relevant than the important one we could be doing. This advice comes from the Irish College of GPs (ICGP 1991):

- Work smarter not harder.
- Develop a sense of time (*see* Appendix to Chapter 6).
- Plan ahead:
  - jobs that must be done today
  - jobs that I can delegate
  - jobs that should be done today
  - jobs that can wait
  - jobs that will never be done.
- Prioritise:
  - urgent, important – do it now
  - non-urgent, important – assign time but do it asap
  - urgent, unimportant – do it next? (perhaps!)
  - non-important, non-urgent – only do if time permits (if at all).
- Identify your best times: use them productively (including for personal time). This may include quiet times to think or read, times when interruptions are unlikely, etc.

- Capitalise on marginal time: e.g. read when travelling, keep short jobs to hand for short time gaps.
- Set deadlines and finish what you start.
- Learn to say no.
- Learn to delegate.
- Use the telephone.
- Keep meetings to a minimum, keep them short and to a time plan.
- Learn to see problems as good – they would find you anyway!
- Minimise interruptions but plan for the inevitable ones.

The following advice can help manage the paperwork mountain:

- Use an in/out tray.
- All mail should come via the in tray to make prioritisation easier.
- Keep this tray empty – it is a mailbox only.
- Put as much as possible in the out tray or bin.
- Try not to handle the same piece of paper twice, i.e. whatever you're going to do, do it now.
- Sort large piles of paperwork on the 'three-pile system', i.e.
  - pile 1 – I must read this
  - pile 2 – I should read this
  - pile 3 – I don't really need to read this.
  Throw pile 3 away and try and repeat the process with pile 2 until you are left with the minimum you are happy about.
- Consider a 'layered' filing system, i.e. a number of trays on your desk perhaps labelled:
  - tray 1 – do today
  - tray 2 – do this week
  - tray 3 – do sometime
  - tray 4 – projects.
  Aim to keep tray 1 clear. Review the second daily and the third when you have time. If any paperwork

remains unactioned for more than a week reconsider if it should be there at all.

► Diary use: use your diary to record anything you would like to remember, but might forget – not just appointments but patients you are particularly worried about or questions that occur to you (Could I learn to excise a chalazion? How often do other people do U&Es in patients on ACEIs?). If you get into this habit and review your diary on a daily basis then your mind does not carry these thoughts and worries around all day and they are not lost forever. If you get to the entry in the diary and feel unmoved to action then put a line through the entry and move on. It also tends to be a lot tidier that 20 Post-its stuck on your desk!

Problem-solving methods

A number of approaches to problem analysis and ways of producing change were mentioned by trainers. These vary from the short acronym to the in-depth psycho-analytical tool. Trainers will have to consider the depth of approach the particular registrar and particular problem require.

Action planning

This is a three-step process to encourage realistic goals for change.

► Step 1: use Figure 7.1 to make sure you are not in the 'swamp' i.e. the change you hope to achieve is within your sphere of influence.
► Step 2: be specific, i.e. define what you want to achieve and how to achieve it.
► Step 3: ask Why? Who? When? Where? How? What?

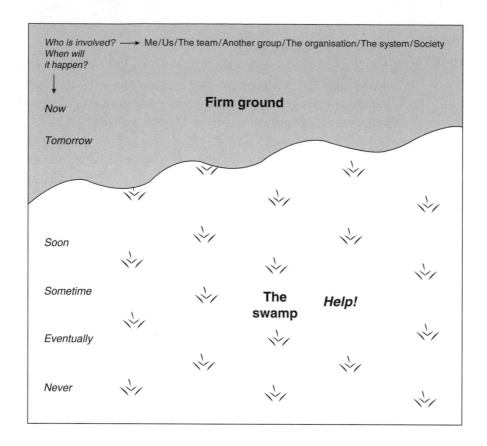

Figure 7.1: Management: spheres of influence.

GROW, FRAME and SMART

A number of short acronyms exist to help the trainer structure brief interactions where change is sought by the learner. Three of these are described below.

GROW – this technique is really designed for the 15–30-minute interaction with a learner to help them find a way forward with a problem.

G goals   What would you like to achieve in this session?

What needs to happen for you to achieve your aim?

Will this be of real value to you?

Is it a realistic aim?

R reality   What is happening now? How often? When does it happen?

Is this an accurate assessment?

What effect does this have?

What other factors are relevant?

Who else is involved? What is their perception?

What have you tried so far? (encouraging self-assessment)

O options   What can you do? (all options)

Who or what could help?

Would you like suggestions?

Which options interest you most? Why?

What are the pros and cons here?

Rate the options 1–10 on practicality.

Would you like to choose one option now?

W wrap up   What are the next steps?

When will you take them?

What might hinder your plans?

What support do you need? How and when will you get it?

How will you know you have achieved your goals?

FRAME – this can be a useful aide-mémoire for planning educational objectives for both learners and trainers.

F	few	Set one or only a few goals
R	realistic	Make the goals achievable
A	agree	If the process involves others enlist their support and agreement
M	measurable	Make sure you will know when the goal is achieved
E	explicit	Try to exclude hidden agendas and keep the process open

SMART – this is very similar to the FRAME technique. It stresses relevance and timing, which may be more appropriate for some registrars.

S	specific	Set a specific objective
M	measurable	Make it measurable
A	attainable	Make it attainable
R	relevant	Make it relevant
T	timed	Time frame the process

Navigation

This is a series of three questions to ask when you set off on the 'journey' of change. Each question contains a number of secondary elements.

1 Where am I/we now? How did we get here? Did the experience teach us anything?
2 Where do I/we want to be? What are our real priorities and how do they fit with this goal? Why do we want to go there? Who is involved?

3 How am I/we going to get there? What will help us? What will hinder us? What routes are possible? With what implications? How will we know we've arrived? (Will we arrive or overshoot?)

POSSEER exercise

This is an exercise in assessing the opportunity for change and helping a person to identify a path forward. You work through the ill-defined problem or goal using the acronym shown below.

P positive	Make sure the goal is stated on positive terms, i.e. 'I'm always late' becomes 'I want to be on time'.
O owned	Define what is in the person's power to achieve, i.e. if you are always late because there is no public transport then you can't catch an earlier bus.
S specific	Define the how, what, where, when and who.
S size	Make it a balance between possibility and challenge, i.e. not too small or too big.
E evidence	How will it be evident the change has occurred? This needs to be explicit.
E ecology	How will the change fit into the person's wider existence?
R resources	Are the tools for the job available?

The aim is to leave the person feeling that the goal is achievable in a practical sense and therefore motivate them to go for it. The facilitator should be able to get an 'acceptance set' (*see* Chapter 2) in response to the question 'are you going to do that then?' at the end of the exercise

Cognitive therapy

The roots of cognitive therapy probably lie in the Socratic style of teaching. Socrates is purported to have helped an uneducated slave prove Pythagoras' theorem simply by asking questions. He achieved this by encouraging the learner to critically examine their own observations, thoughts, feelings and experiences and to use new insights to build self-constructed concepts on secure foundations. Easy, eh! The cognitive therapy model aims to make this process accessible to the rest of us. For example, let us assume a registrar's surgeries always run very late. A jointly developed analysis of the situation may be as shown in Figure 7.2.

The behaviours, moods, thoughts and physical feelings are analysed and placed on the framework as shown in Figure 7.2. The trainer facilitates this process by bringing out unconscious or hidden elements. The framework can then be used to develop strategies for change, which can range from simple symptom management (relaxation techniques) to behavioural change (book patients at 20-minute intervals for now and have some sessions on consultation skills) and even to looking at value systems (What is 'good' medicine? Who has first call on your time?). It is not suggested that every problem needs this in-depth approach although it does seem a useful way to identify the causes, effects and possible solution areas when change is necessary.

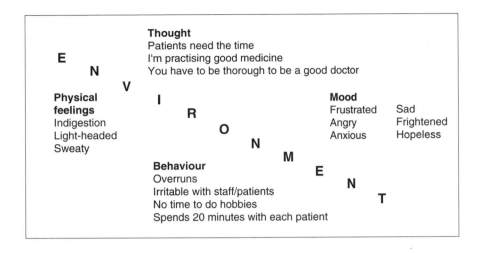

Figure 7.2: Cognitive behavioural theory model.

Logical levels exercise

This is an exercise that can be done with pen and paper (perhaps for the theorist) or physically 'hopping' on a series of cards (for the activist). It asserts that a problem or perceived need for change can be looked at on a number of levels.

- Level 1   What is the problem?
- Level 2   What do I feel about the problem?
- Level 3   What do I think about the problem?
- Level 4   What values do I have around this issue?
- Level 5   What beliefs underpin my values?

The registrar is taken through this process by considering a number of questions – these can be written on cards and placed on the floor. The registrar hops from one question to the next describing their responses at each station.

Q1	Where are you?	(scene setting)
Q2	What is the problem/area for change?	(clarifying goal)
Q3	How do you feel about this?	(feelings)
Q4	What are you thinking about this?	(thoughts)
Q5	What do these thoughts mean?	(interpretation)
Q6	Why do you believe they mean this?	(values)
Q7	Who are you?	(personal comfort/role)
Q8	Are you comfortable with your beliefs?	(beliefs)
Q9	Is change still necessary?	(check problem still real)
Q10	Name a specific change you can make?	(identify change)

Enough insight into the problem or need for change may develop at any question level and the process can stop at this point. If the registrar completes the process they can run back through the questions (starting at Q1) imagining the change has occurred. This can help check that the proposed change feels appropriate.

SWOT analysis

The SWOT technique describes a tool designed to facilitate the analysis of a situation where no clear-cut solution or way forward exists. The situation is analysed under the four headings:

▸ **S**trengths
▸ **W**eaknesses
▸ **O**pportunities
▸ **T**hreats.

The process illustrates the links between threats and opportunities, strengths and weaknesses and encourages all parties to contribute to an overall picture. Hopefully a more balanced decision emerges.

Some thoughts on change

Why is change so difficult to achieve sometimes and so automatic at others? Three areas shed some light on this question.

A Habits: we are creatures of habit and once we have developed a pattern of behaviour we derive security from this and resist losing it.

B Externalisations: if we perceive that an external force has control we are often slow to recognise our own control (i.e. the locus of control theory).

C Self-disciplines: even if we perceive the need for change it requires motivation and drive to achieve it.

The 'four fears' often act as additional blocks to change:

► fear of failure
► fear of change (the 'devil I know' syndrome)
► fear of self-confrontation/self-exposure
► fear of success.

These ideas can be helpful in the analysis of difficult situations.

Motivation

Many trainers feel that high motivation is one of the key elements of successful training. Maslow's scale (with

Neighbour's modification) and Glasser's table provide some insights in this area (*see* Introduction to Chapter 4). The rank ordering scale (*see* Appendix A) is a practical tool to help analyse driving forces. What other ways do trainers use to look at the problem of motivation? The two cycles of demotivation are shown in Figures 7.3 and 7.4.

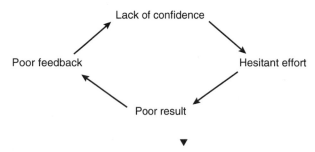

Figure 7.3: Negative cycle of demotivation.

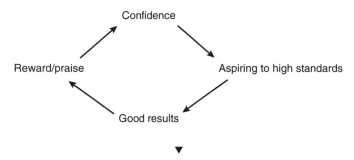

Figure 7.4: Positive cycle of demotivation.

If the registrar is within the negative cycle of de-motivation the trainer can highlight the problem and work on confidence building, i.e. jointly select an area where good performance can be anticipated (everyone has some good potential skills), construct a plan and ensure plenty of feedback. If the registrar is in the positive cycle of demotivation it is usually a lack of reward or praise that is the problem. Doctors are notoriously poor at providing positive feedback. A simple 'well done' or acknowledgement of patient satisfaction can have an enormous effect.

In the *BJGP* (July 1998) Miller *et al.* looked specifically at motivation to learn in GPs. They propose a developmental view of learning motivations. A simplification of this approach is summarised in Table 7.1. This model encourages us to accept that different motivators are at work in different learners. It can help us to appreciate and perhaps harness the registrar's motivators and encourages the concept of developing his or her motivations by trying to move the learner towards the right of the scale. This involves stimulating individual development, perhaps by raising awareness of professional values and the breadth of general practice. Providing appropriate role models is also highlighted.

The motivating skills questionnaire can provide trainers with some insight into their own motivating skills. The questionnaire is designed to assess a person's managerial skill in motivating others. It can act as an interesting stimulus to discussion in this area. It is described in detail in the Appendix at the end of this chapter.

Table 7.1: A developmental view of motivation to learn in GPs

Stages	Motivators	Type of learner
Innate	Curiosity Altruism	Global unfocused
Early learning	Global unfocused Role models	Superficial
Socialisation	Peer pressure	Deep
Professionalisation	Professional values Reputation Security Job satisfaction	Strategic
Independence	Pragmatism	Tactical

The 'what' of management

In response to the comments of many newly vocationally trained GPs (who express anxieties about their training in this area), some trainers use a list of management areas for the registrar to consider. The list aims to open the registrar's eyes to the scope of the management role to enable him or her to define his or her own learning objectives. A sample list is shown in the Appendix to this chapter. The Appendix also contains an in-depth look at the insurance element of running a practice. This can be a useful tool for discussion and tends to open a registrar's perspective of practice management.

Teams

The need to function within a team is an essential element of modern general practice. Registrars need to be suitably equipped to achieve this. The following sections offer resources to stimulate thought in this area. The use of Belbin's team style inventory and the assertion rights questionnaire are described in Chapter 3.

Characteristics of effective teams

This is a list of the ideal team components for discussion:

- ► **Vision and common purpose** – the team members know why the team exists. They have clear objectives and a shared vision. They focus on results and are good at setting priorities and making decisions.
- ► **Communication** – this is vital, open and honest. Feedback is valued and conflict resolved. Team members listen, say what they think and respect others' views. Team members are able to challenge each other with no hidden agendas.

- **Trust and respect** – all team members are valued and supported as valid contributors to the whole performance.
- **Shared leadership** – leadership is not based on status or position. The formal leader is a coach and mentor. The appropriate leader(s) emerges and all team members take responsibility for decisions. When necessary a leader to take quick decisions emerges. Team members are empowered to take part in decision making where appropriate.
- **Procedural** – the team develops policies and rules designed to help achieve goals. The team is efficient at gathering information, mustering resources, organising and evaluating. Creativity, innovation and good risk assessment are all valued.
- **Flexibility and adaptability** – the team sees change as an opportunity more than a threat. The team is constantly looking to improve processes and tends to delegate this to appropriate members.
- **Team roles** – the team recognises different strengths in different members and sees this as a resource to use and learn from. The team looks for gaps in its function and seeks to remedy these by training, recruitment or outside resource use.
- **Learning** – the team takes measured risks and learns from mistakes. There is an expectation of individual growth and an encouragement of questions. They expect learning opportunities in all situations. Actions are considered, agreed and evaluated. New learning produces appropriate change.

Behaviours seen in effective teams

This list can look superficially similar to the one above, but is looking at the same elements from a behavioural point of view. This allows more analysis of where problems might lie and also points towards solutions. It has a more pragmatic feel to it than the more theoretical list of ideals above.

- ▶ **Clear goals**
  - team roles are clarified (job descriptions, titles, areas of responsibility)
  - acceptable differences are defined (codes of conduct, disciplinary codes, dress codes, contracts)
  - values are discussed and consensus reached (meeting forums, mission statements).
- ▶ **Support and trust**
  - feelings are recognised and dealt with (feedback systems, support networks)
  - people display empathy, respect and are genuine (no cliques, no jealousies, people choose to spend time and talk together at and across all levels of the organisation)
  - individual worries are shared in a supportive manner.
- ▶ **Communication**
  - honest feedback is given sensitively (positive and negative) to everyone (appraisals, reward systems)
  - people communicate well person to person.
- ▶ **Conflict**
  - conflicts are seen as inevitable and sources of growth
  - conflicts are dealt with rapidly
  - all parties are encouraged to be assertive
  - discussions are 'solution-based' and people are not blamed
  - attempts are made to minimise areas of conflict.
- ▶ **Procedures**
  - there are clear procedures that are helpful (protocols, policies)
  - delegation is explicit and empowering
  - meetings are actively managed (agendas, times, minutes, actions).

▶ **Leadership**
- the leadership is constructive and uses the strengths of the team.

▶ **Evaluation**
- the team reviews its progress (audits, reports, use of data)
- this process is focused on producing a better result.

▶ **Individual development**
- the team aims to promote improvement in the performance of all members (appraisals, training, courses, promotion).

▶ **Perspective**
- the team looks both inwards and outwards to build relationships (other commitments, links to other bodies, use of outside resources).

Assertiveness

Assertiveness rights questionnaire

Assertiveness is seen as one of the important elements of the effective team member. Many individuals' assertiveness skills are either non-existent or linked to an aggressive approach. This not only reduces their effectiveness but produces collateral damage as it offends others or leaves them frustrated. The assertion rights questionnaire is described in Chapter 3. This enables the trainer to look at this emotive area through the 'third party' of the questionnaire. In practice, this tends to make the exercise less threatening. The result produces a combination of the 'OK' and 'not OK' scenarios:

▶ **I'm OK, you're OK, assertive behaviour, win–win**
We value each other and ourselves, listen to each other and share our thoughts and feelings honestly.

▶ **I'm not OK, you're OK, passive behaviour, lose–win**

I think you embody what I am not and although I respect you I don't think you really want to hear what I have to say. It's easier to keep quiet and do what you want me to because I want you to like me and I don't feel equal to you.

▶ **I'm OK, you're not OK, aggressive behaviour, win–lose**

I think I know better and am more important than you. I may interrupt and ignore you. I don't really need to make much effort to let you have what you're entitled to.

▶ **I'm not OK, you're not OK, indirect aggression, lose–lose**

I don't have much faith in you, or myself. I feel at war with you but would not tell you that. I have little self-respect so I avoid issues, preferring to use insincere praise and flattery to try and get my way. I will try and undermine you behind your back.

Assertiveness 'bill of rights'

This is a simple list of individual rights. A discussion or even a rank ordering of this list can be a useful tool for identifying values and attitudes in this area. Trainers have found this useful when they have identified potential problems in registrars.

▶ To be treated with respect as a capable and equal human being.
▶ To have and express my own feelings, values and opinions without having to justify or apologise for them.
▶ To be listened to seriously.
▶ To set my own priorities and state my own needs and be myself – not what others want or expect me to be.

- To say yes or no for myself without guilt.
- To have the right to make mistakes and to change my mind sometimes.
- To ask for what I want, accepting that I may not always get it.
- To say I don't understand.
- To choose not to be assertive.

Assertiveness training

These simple techniques can be offered to the registrar with problems:

- Ownership – use 'I' statements, i.e. I think, I want.
- Don't ramble – try and state your words concisely and clearly.
- Ask questions – ask open questions to establish other people's opinions, i.e. I'm not sure about this.
- Listen – learn to actively listen at all times.
- Involvement – try to reduce the emotional content in both yourself and others when being assertive, i.e. I'm not trying to make you angry; I'm sorry if this upsets you but we do need to sort it out.
- Say what you want.
- Set limits – so you can't be manipulated.
- 'Broken record' technique – keep repeating your view if you are feeling ignored.

Leadership

The true leader is always led

Jung

Many people would suggest that an awareness of leadership skills is essential for the GP. The following lists can provide a basis for discussion.

1 Questions?
   - Name four leaders. Were they successful? What skills did they possess? (Try it on Hitler and Churchill or politicians or sportsmen)
   - Think of someone you have had personal contact with as a leader? Why were you impressed?
   - What are the skills the perfect leader would have?
   - How does someone acquire these skills?
   - Where have you seen effective/less effective leadership in the practice?
2 Good leadership is characterised by:
   - continuity
   - willingness to invest time
   - a vision of the goal
   - ability to motivate others
   - a belief in the goal
   - an overall perception of the situation
   - energy and enthusiasm
   - ability to see and get the best from others.
3 The functions of a leader include:
   - establishing, communicating and clarifying goals
   - motivating
   - establishing processes
   - setting standards
   - acting as a role model (*see* Table 3.1)
   - encouraging and rewarding
   - monitoring and evaluating
   - maximising resource efficiency
   - providing feedback
   - highlighting foreseeable problems.

Delegation

Effective management has been defined as 'performing tasks through others'. If this is true then delegation is a core skill for GPs. This section looks at the use of delegation as a teaching tool and describes some thoughts on delegation that may help in tutorial design.

Delegation as a teaching tool – the skill/will matrix

Trainers need to know how to delegate, when to delegate and how to facilitate the development of delegation skills in learners (Landsberg 1997). Delegation is sometimes desirable but not advisable. The skill/will matrix is an interesting way of analysing this situation. Figure 7.5 illustrates this technique. The trainer must form an opinion of the registrar's skill level and motivation for a particular aspect of training. The matrix then suggests appropriate training techniques to improve the probability that learning will occur.

The term coaching is defined in Chapter 6. Directive coaching commits the trainer to two tasks: first, the provision of a safe, structured and controlled environment for learning; and second, the duty to analyse and stimulate motivation. Delegative coaching involves a more hands-off approach to the high achiever while remaining available for feedback and consultation. The aim is to develop the learner's skills and stimulate their motivation to allow the delegative style. This matrix has the potential to help trainers and registrars design appropriate educational experiences.

HIGH WILL	High skill	Deficient skill
	Peak performer	*Enthusiastic beginner*
METHOD	**Delegative coaching**	**Supervisory coaching**
	• Help to set objectives (not methods)	• Provide structure
	• Praise (not ignore)	• Control and supervise closely
	• Devolve decision making	• Use informative questions
	• Use interpretative questions	• Praise/listen and facilitate
	• Increase awareness of potential	• Safety net to allow mistakes–be slow to chide
LOW WILL	*Reluctant contributor*	*Disillusioned learner*
METHOD	**Excite/motivate/supportive coaching**	**Directive coaching**
	• Analyse motivation	• Look at motivation
	• Provide stimulation	• Look at ability
	• Look for personal problems	• Clear communication lines
	• Praise, listen and facilitate	• Develop a path forwards
		• Provide positive feedback opportunities (i.e. play to strengths)
		• Control, supervise and structure

▼

Figure 7.5: Skill/will matrix.

Teaching delegation skills

Many registrars have to adapt to the process of delegation in the practice with little awareness of the principles. The following points may help open this area up in a tutorial.

What are the purposes of delegation:

- ► to deal with the task effectively *and* efficiently?
- ► to ensure optimum use of capacity?
- ► to free up the delegator to allow them to use time for more important tasks?
- ► to stimulate staff and increase their competencies?
- ► to create an atmosphere of achievement and responsibility?
- ► sometimes to increase financial rewards?

It should *not*:

► create a feeling of dumping on staff
► lower standards
► overload staff.

Why don't people delegate more? There are a number of possible reasons listed below. Sometimes it is simply that we are 'intimidated by talent' as one manager put it.

► It upsets one's ego (no one else can do it can they?).
► Anxiety about mistakes (I'm the only one who doesn't make mistakes).
► Anxiety about the process (my way is the only way).
► Fear of loss of control (I'm the boss).
► Desire for perfection (no one else will do it as well as I can).
► Lack of confidence in others (they are all useless).
► False sense of efficiency (I can do everything anyway).

So what about the principles of good delegation? Box 7.1 shows the 'nine-point guide to perfect delegation'. Point 5 involves the completed staffwork concept. This was a tool described by Napoleon Bonaparte. If there was a problem in the army and his general asked for a solution then he was dismissed. If the general had analysed the situation and developed the options he could stay, i.e. the delegator should expect to advise and not sort things out themselves.

> **Box 7.1: The nine-point guide to perfect delegation**
>
> 1 Select the right person
> 2 Give them explicit instructions
> 3 Provide them with the tools for the job
> 4 Assign a task and an outcome (but not *exactly* how to do it)
> 5 Use the completed staffwork system
> 6 Don't attach strings (i.e. allow them to think and develop)
> 7 Resist upward delegation (e.g. 'How did you want me to do this?')
> 8 Agree a deadline
> 9 Follow through (i.e. feedback and monitor)

When you delegate to someone make sure you give them the responsibility that goes with the task, the authority to do it and the accountability for the result. Where possible it is helpful to delegate an area of management to the registrar. Examples have included a role in the winter flu vaccination campaign, the purchase of a piece of equipment, the writing and implementation of a new policy, etc. The audit project has potential in this area.

The five delegation zones

- ▶ Zone 1 – tasks that cannot be delegated.
- ▶ Zone 2 – tasks that the delegator should deal with. These should only really be delegated if professionally acceptable and when the trainer is under extreme time pressure or if the delegation is more in the form of assistance, i.e. the responsibility remains with the delegator.
- ▶ Zone 3 – tasks that could be delegated. The delegator has the most appropriate skills but other staff could do this with support and training.

▸ Zone 4 – tasks that should be delegated. Other staff have the skills to do this already.

▸ Zone 5 – tasks that must be delegated. These are the tasks that the delegator may have process knowledge of but does not possess the skills to perform.

It can be an interesting exercise to go through a surgery looking at which zone the various tasks completed fall into. This can be particularly relevant to the registrar who runs very late or fails to use the PHCT effectively.

Other points to note

Relationship between performance and satisfaction

Figure 7.6 illustrates the relationship in the managerial environment between performance and satisfaction. This has implications for the training environment. Achieving a balance between the two elements of performance pressure and need for satisfaction can be difficult. We must try and aim to work in the integrative arena.

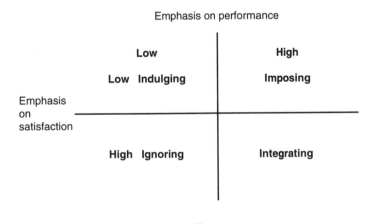

Figure 7.6: Performance and satisfaction in the working/learning environment.

Equation of task performance

If the trainer or registrar are armchair mathematicians or have strong theorist tendencies then they may find Maier and Lawler's formulae food for thought:

performance = ability × motivation (effort)
ability = aptitude × training × resources
motivation = desire × commitment.

Summary comments

Postgraduate training is all about adult education. The responsibility for learning and changing lie with the registrar. It may be helpful to look at the principles of the adult learning process, which are shown in Box 7.2.

Box 7.2: Principles of adult learning

The most effective learning occurs when:

- a good learner/facilitator (not teacher!) relationship exists
- adults select their own learning experiences (self-directed)
- there is an environment where new skills can be practised readily
- the learner's past experience/learning is taken into account
- the learner's learning style is taken into account
- there are opportunities for the learner to pass on his or her own wisdom
- there is a non-threatening environment
- there is a good available standard the learner can use to assess himself or herself by
- the learner can assess his or her own progress towards personal goals.

Adult learners bring expectations, intentions, life skills and real life demands to the learning environment and trainers need to recognise these. Trainers need to keep the learning process focused on its relevant context, i.e. clinical teaching should involve clinical material, and management teaching should involve management material. This is emphasised because much of this section has described techniques that seem a little distant from the real world. They must be seen as complementary techniques or even diagnostic techniques. The bulk of management training should involve placing the registrar in management scenarios for experiential learning. Many of the techniques described increase the potential for learning and change.

Appendix to Chapter 7

The 'what' of management

In-depth insurance analysis

This is an in-depth pnemonic to use as a tool to raise awareness of the complexity of practice management by looking at one area – the insurance aspects of practice.

I	Insure in everyone's sight	Impossible to self-insure
	If it can go wrong it will	Insure with professionals
	Insurance products do change	Insist on regular reviews/requotes
	Instigate actions to reduce risk	Insist premiums are itemised
N	Never fail to report incidences	Never fail to disclose
	Never underinsure	New circumstances must be notified
	Never underestimate exposure	Never be complacent
S	Sleep at night	Security of policies and documents
	Stage payments	Spouse protection
	Staff risks – fraud/indemnity	Sessional staff cover
	Stamp duties – hidden charges	Structure of practice can affect cover
	Special areas – product liability	
U	Use a valuer for building insurance	Use an insurance broker
	Unforced entry may not be covered	Under statutory obligations – public liability

R Read the policy
Report claims promptly
in writing
Report events

Risk assessment – do one
Review coverage regularly
Rental properties are
special considerations

E Expect explanation of
policy
External party exposure
Exposure professionally
Excess amounts

Ensure you know the
exclusions
Expect only one insurer
to pay out
Extensions to policies
Earnings – loss of

Major areas to cover:

- ► buildings and fixtures
- ► contents
- ► computers – including data reinstatement
- ► loss of earnings
- ► house and contents
- ► loss of life
- ► motor vehicles
- ► public liability
- ► product liability
- ► professional liability
- ► staff liability
- ► special events
- ► machinery breakdown.

The 'what' of management list

Practice organisation

This document is designed to raise an awareness of practice management in registrars. You should have a passing acquaintance with the following documents:

- ► Statement of Fees and Allowances (the Red Book)
- ► terms and conditions of employment
- ► a practice management textbook.

The following list is intended as a template to help you gather the relevant information.

- ► **Staffing**
  - – 'Hiring and firing', i.e. job descriptions/contracts/ legal requirements and employment
  - – Law/disciplinary procedures/pay and tax/staff acquisition/training and
  - – Qualifications/assessment and development/reimbursements/posts in practice.
- ► **Partnership**
  - – Sorts of job available (locum/assistant/salaried/part-time/retainer/share, etc.)
  - – Partnership agreements
  - – Selection processes
  - – Common pitfalls/survival techniques
  - – Single-handed posts.
- ► **Finances**
  - – Money in: HA/private work/outside commitments/ entrepreneurial
  - – Money out
  - – Reimbursements
  - – Personal aspects: salary/tax/accountancy, etc.
  - – Capital costs: buildings/equipment/cost rent scheme
  - – Insurance.
- ► **Drugs**
  - – Dispensing/personally administered items
  - – PACT

- IPAs
- Incentive schemes.
▶ **Primary care groups/trusts**
- Principles
- Main practical elements, i.e. budget setting/budget components/contracts/savings/governance
- Alternatives systems.
▶ **Administration**
- Computing: potential uses/links/PCG/targets/data manipulation, etc.
- Paperwork: forms/returns/in-house systems/medical record systems.
▶ **Advertisement**
- 'Selling' the practice/viability and growth
- Relationship with outside agencies/reps, etc.
- Relationship with HA/hospitals/LMC/local trusts, etc.
▶ **IT**
- Computers in the surgery/decision support systems/patient education
- Computers in management
- External links (HA/hospitals/internet/Prodigy/other).
▶ **Other**
- Add any more that occur to you.

The motivating skills questionnaire

One of the most important aspects of change is understanding motivation. How good are we at motivating others?

The following questionnaire provides a method of looking at our motivational skills. Answer the following questions using the rating scale below:

1 strongly disagree	2 disagree	3 slightly disagree
4 slightly agree	5 agree	6 strongly agree

Imagine that you are supervising the work of a registrar:

Score

1 If my registrar's performance is poor or inefficient the first thing I would do is to check whether they had the skills, knowledge and tools to do the work, THEN I would worry about motivation ————

2 I would establish the standards I expect my registrar to achieve ————

3 If necessary I would offer to provide training and would not take over the problem myself ————

4 I would be straightforward in providing feedback of how he/she is doing and his/her chances of securing a good post after training ————

5 I always attempt to find ways of rewarding exceptional performance ————

6 If it came to having to discipline the registrar I would identify the problem, describe its consequences and explain how it should be corrected ————

Score

7 I try to make work both interesting and
   rewarding   ———

8 I try to match the rewards to the person
   when the job is done well   ———

9 I make sure that the person feels fairly
   and equitably treated   ———

10 I make sure that the person gets timely
   feedback from those affected by their
   performance   ———

11 I attempt to find the reasons for poor
   performance before taking any remedial
   action   ———

12 I always help the person to set targets
   that are challenging, specific and
   timebound   ———

13 Only as a last resort do I attempt to
   remove or fire someone   ———

14 Whenever possible I make sure valued
   rewards are linked to high performance   ———

15 I am very tough when the effort is
   below what is required and I know what
   can be achieved   ———

16 I try to make work more interesting by
   varying the nature of the work and
   modifying tasks to provide variety   ———

17 I try to arrange for teamworking
   wherever possible   ———

18 I make sure that any judgements of
   performance are fair   ———

19 I reward success immediately   ———

20 I always determine if the person has the
   necessary resources and support to
   succeed in the task   ———

Total   ———

Motivating skills questionnaire – scoring guide

To find your score for each skill area simply add up the numbers for the relevant questions.

Skill area	*Question No.*	*Score*
Diagnosing performance problems	1, 11	
Establishing expectations and goal setting	2, 12	
Facilitating performance (enhancing ability)	3, 13, 20	
Linking performance to reward and discipline	5, 6, 14, 15	
Using salient internal and external incentives	7, 8, 16, 17	
Distributing rewards equitably	9, 18	
Providing timely feedback	4, 10, 19	
Total		_____

- ▸ Maximum score 120
- ▸ 500 business school students:
  - $>$101 top quartile
  - 94–101 second quartile
  - 85–93 third quartile
  - $<$84 bottom quartile

Time management diary

This is a tool to facilitate the analysis of a person's use of time. The diary can be kept for a week or a day (although a 'typical' day should be chosen). Record every hour your current activity. Break this down into the following areas, using the diary to remind you of the actual content of each hour:

- appointments in the surgery
- travelling time
- time seeing patients in their own home
- leisure time
- sleep
- eating
- paperwork
- meetings
- reading
- other.

Produce a pie chart of the time period.

Hour	Activity	Comment
0100		
0200		
0300		
0400		
0500		
0600		
0700		
0800		
0900		
1000		
1100		
1200		
1300		

Hour	Activity	Comment
1400		
1500		
1600		
1700		
1800		
1900		
2000		
2100		
2200		
2300		
2400		

CHAPTER 8

Assessment: how do trainers make use of the assessment process?

'I dunno,' said Arthur, 'I forget what I was taught, I only remember what I've learnt'

TH White

Introduction

The theme of assessment runs through the whole of the educational process and this theme has been mentioned many times already. This chapter looks specifically at how trainers use the formative, summative and MRCGP processes to augment learning.

Formative assessment

The concept of formative assessment is alien to many registrars. It can be helpful to discuss the differences between formative and summative assessment early on, perhaps using the educational cycle illustration (*see* Chapter 6). Trainers felt the following points were important:

► **Atmosphere** – get the relationship between trainer and registrar *right*. Chapter 5 discusses features of this point.

▶ **Feedback** – the principles of positive feedback are covered in Chapter 5. The following points were emphasised by trainers:
  – provide positive feedback regarding assessment
  – encourage feedback *from* the registrar to the trainer
  – view feedback as a *gift*, i.e. choose it carefully, wrap it appropriately, give it at the right time, give it openly
  – remember Pendleton's rules (*see* Chapter 2)
  – provide and receive feedback regularly, honestly and with humility and confidentiality
  – always check the evidence base for your feedback
  – make a note of particularly good work to bring up when appropriate; 'be quick to praise and slow to chide'.

▶ **Process**
  – start this early
  – when filling in analogue scales the registrar and trainer can do this independently and compare the results. Often the areas of greatest difference are the ones to discuss
  – use the process to demonstrate change (hopefully improvement!)
  – consider encouraging the registrar to keep a log diary
  – consider the following ways of obtaining evidence for assessment:
    (i) feedback from PHCT (often confirms the trainer's concerns)
    (ii) note reviews
    (iii) MCQs
    (iv) patients' views (by asking other doctors in the practice usually)
    (v) a formal process (e.g. MCQ, MEQ, joint surgery/visits or video)
    (vi) review referrals/prescriptions.

These pointers can help trainers to optimise their use of the opportunities available in the formative assessment process.

Summative assessment

Currently, all registrars have to complete summative assessment. This involves four components. The following sections detail the points trainers feel are important in coping with these components. The most consistent point was to start the process early and certainly discuss this in the first week or two.

The written component

The UKCRA written component of summative assessment

The registrar has to perform an audit. All deaneries supply the registrars with the proforma which involves a series of questions to be answered (*see* Appendix to this chapter). On the face of it the process looks simple and yet a significant number are 'referred', i.e. have to be resubmitted. Most then pass but the resubmission process is at least time-consuming and at worst very upsetting. So why does this happen? The main reasons for referral seem to be:

▸ too complex an audit and the registrar has got lost in the 'process'
▸ too few patients (try for at least 20–100)
▸ standards are set inappropriately (often no GP references)
▸ the terms 'standards' and 'criteria' are demonstrably misunderstood
▸ no change seems possible as an outcome
▸ there is no evidence of any teamwork.

With these points in mind trainers offered the following advice:

▸ **Structure**
  – provide a file of examples (MAAG can help, keep previous registrar's audits, show your own audits)

- teach the terminology (*see* Appendix to this chapter)
- stimulate the registrar to produce ideas (the ideas framework, the audit game (*see* Appendix to this chapter)
- show them the marking schedule (*see* Appendix to this chapter)
- emphasise (i) value of process
  (ii) KISS (Keep It Short and Simple), i.e. ask one question
  (iii) do it early
  (iv) it is easy
  (v) the best idea for the audit is their own idea.

▶ **Process**
- give the registrar protected time
- encourage him or her to discuss the problems with their peers, you or anyone!
- regularly review progress and reiterate submission deadline
- advise him or her to use the computer for data collection where possible
- suggest the use of outside advice where necessary (MAAG, Royal Colleges, specialists, etc.)
- suggest he or she uses GP references as much as possible and certainly if a standard is set
- suggest he or she tries to complete the cycle or at least consider how it would be completed
- make sure some change is possible
- make sure he or she uses the staff in some meaningful way (even if only to get notes out, etc.) and make it explicit in the submission
- make sure their presentation is 'assessor friendly', i.e. clear text, tables, graphs, etc.
- ANSWER the questions set, preferably on the form supplied
- DON'T PANIC – very few people fail on this element alone.

Trainers suggested the following resources be considered:

► delegate to an informed and interested partner (usually the 'auditor')
► MAAG
► find out your local summative assessment written submission first line assessor and ask for advice
► discuss the problems at the trainers' workshops
► and try to avoid statisticians!

The Appendix to this chapter contains a short summary of audit theory that clarifies some of the points registrars struggle with.

The Yorkshire Marking Schedule for Written Submission

After three years of development in Yorkshire, this method of testing the written skills of summative assessment was approved by the JCPTGP. It differs from the UKCRA method because it allows the registrar to submit surveys, notes, reviews, case studies, research reports and audits. It is available nationally but most deaneries continue to use the UKCRA method of assessment.

The Summative Assessment MCQ

Trainers see this as a low hurdle that registrars should jump easily and quickly – certainly within the first three months of the year. These points were put forward:

► make sure the registrar gets the date of the MCQ firmly in mind
► use book-based (*see* Chapter 11) or PEP-based (*see* Chapter 3) material to boost confidence and identify needs.

One trainer suggested a neat reminder of the value of a diary in the form of the following equation:

$$WD_{LB} + LU_{BB} = K$$

(write down in little book plus look up in big book equals knowledge)

The registrar can also be reminded that the MRCGP MCQ provides exemption from this element of summative assessment (if they pass!).

The Trainer's Report

A copy of the trainer's report is reproduced in the Appendix to this chapter. Many trainers feel comparatively unprepared for this element of summative assessment. The report is highly detailed, calls for specific evidence and involves assessing very basic clinical skills as well as the more subtle areas of general practice. Many of the questions posed are poorly defined and it is far from clear how much detail is required.

With all this in mind, trainers advised:

▸ Start this early – week one!
▸ Try and use it formatively, i.e. openly discussing it with the registrar and using it to set objectives.
▸ Use the PHCT where necessary (i.e. the nurse to tell you about PV examination, etc.).
▸ Use his or her CV and discussion to cover the basics (consider checking with references from consultants).
▸ Use video and joint surgeries/visits – record the dates and competencies demonstrated.
▸ Go over the report as a trainers' workshop exercise.
▸ Identify areas of concern early and work on them.
▸ A diary of educational experience kept by the registrar *and* a diary of the educational process kept by the trainer are invaluable.
▸ Set time aside to fill it in.
▸ Put it somewhere prominent to remind everyone to look at it regularly.
▸ Consider programming review of it (perhaps even once a week).

There are a range of options to consider when completing the form. Some trainers adopt the minimalist approach and 'tick' the boxes. Others are concerned the form may come back to haunt them in the future if the registrar's competence is questioned later in their career. One trainer's workshop agreed (using section 10 of the report as an example) on the format illustrated in Box 8.1, with the proviso that if real concerns were apparent the advice above was followed.

Box 8.1: Example of trainer's report

10 The doctor undertakes appropriate examination (including investigation)

Assessment by direct observation of registrar by assessor	Assessment by discussion between registrar and assessor	Assessment by specific methods	Comments
Video sessions on *(with dates)* Joint surgeries on *(with dates)* Practice nurse feedback *(with relevant area)*	Tutorial on investigation *(or other relevant subject)* *(with dates)*	Analysis of use of investigation Past qualifications *(noting relevant ones)*	No apparent problems *(or use this area to add formative assessment comments, i.e. would like to develop slit lamp skills)*

If a trainer feels unable to satisfactorily fill in the report then it is essential that the reasons for this are explicit and evidence to support this reasoning is available. In this situation the regional training practice approval system is likely to consider whether part of the problem lies within the practice. The prudent trainer will have taken the following steps as early in the training process as possible:

- Discuss the problems with the registrar.
- Discuss them with other doctors in the practice.
- Discuss them with your course organiser EARLY.
- Discuss them with your regional advisor.
- Document EVERYTHING.
- Consider keeping evidence (video tapes, notes, etc.).

The video component

Registrars are required to submit a two-hour video tape of consultations for assessment. It is advised this should be completed after about six months in practice. They are allowed to edit this tape and it is submitted with identification and brief clinical details of each patient. The marking schedule is shown in Chapter 2. Deanery general practice departments send guidelines on the submission to all registrars and trainers. Trainers offered the following advice on this element:

- Get the video out early in the year (first week).
- Emphasise the positive aspects of video-taping consultations.
- Get registrars to do lots of video recordings with brief notes made on each consultation (perhaps on an appointment list).
- Suggest the registrar record 'low-pressure' surgeries, i.e. on half-days/Saturday mornings). This reduces the time pressure on them and gets the practice staff into a routine.
- Get the staff to do all the consenting, i.e.:
  - tell patients when they book the appointment it will be recorded
  - get them to sign the form in the waiting room
  - get them to sign again after consulting
  - get them to chase up unsigned forms.

- Use the standard consent forms – remember registrars can use this tape for the MRCGP also, so ensure the right forms are signed.
- Have a video-based tutorial using the marking forms.
- Trainers should always see the final result before submission.
- Registrars should select the cases for the final submission.
- Make sure the clinical comments are helpful. They can even be used to try and show awareness of a problem area in the tape, i.e. perhaps a cue was missed and a comment made on this point.
- Get advice from an assessor if necessary.
- Tell the registrar:
    - remember the basics
    - don't try to be too clever
    - avoid very long (>20 minutes) or short (<5 minutes) consultations. Aim for the 8–15-minute range
    - don't submit a tape of all low-challenge patients
    - consider submitting a tape of one surgery with no editing (many hours can be wasted editing).

MRCGP examination

Trainers have very mixed feelings about the role of the MRCGP examination in the training year. This section does not intend to cover advice for registrars on how to prepare or pass the MRCGP. This is well covered in many books (*see* Chapter 10). This section describes how trainers have sought to use the MRCGP to add to their educational programmes. Many registrars are examination-orientated. They may have openly declared their intention to sit the MRCGP. This group tends to respond well to examination-orientated teaching methods. When a learning need is identified the examination processes can be mimicked to address that need, that is:

▶ From October 2000 a pass in the MRCGP Video Assessment of Consulting Skills is also acceptable for summative assessment purposes.
▶ The registrar consults in a very doctor-centred manner – use the MRCGP video marking grid with emphasis on the patient-centred performance criteria.
▶ The registrar needs to look at team approaches to managing chronic disease – devise an MEQ type question that encompasses this area.
▶ The trainer is concerned that the registrar has difficulty dealing with abortion requests – state that you are going to use an oral-type format used in the exam to look at values and attitudes and use this subject.

This requires a certain familiarity with the examination process but this can be achieved by looking at one of the exam guides.

The following pieces of advice are also offered:

▶ If the registrar is going to sit the examination, advise him or her:
  – to try and prepare in a group
  – to go on an approved course run by examiners (usually 2–5 days)
  – to talk to colleagues who have recently passed the MRCGP
  – to plan their preparation – read one of the MRCGP books
  – to get plenty of exam practice (including oral practice)
  – it is likely to dominate a large section of the year in practice
  – to look carefully at the modular structure.
▶ Tell the registrar to get into the habit of always thinking 'why?'.

The Appendix to this chapter contains a number of tools that trainers have found useful both for examination preparation and in the training year. These are:

- a list of statistical terms for discussion
- critical appraisal skills handout
- READER scheme for critical appraisal
- the 1998 modular MRCGP structure summary.

Assessing the quality of training

Registrars who pass the MRCGP (and possibly summative assessment) provide some evidence of quality of training. Chapter 5 looked at how trainers assess the quality of tutorials. Are trainers using any other methods to assess the quality of their training? Apart from the 'bums on seats' approach suggested by one trainer (and many trainers cannot attract registrars) the following methods were described.

Feedback forms

Deanery documentation

Many deaneries have confidential feedback forms that registrars submit at the end of the year. No trainer admitted to ever having received feedback from this source. An example is included in the Appendix to this chapter.

Registrar end of year report

This asks for a simple list of up to 10 aspects of the year that best met expectations and the 10 that could be improved (*see* Appendix to this chapter).

The trainer rating scales

This set of scales was developed in the Burton-on-Trent area and covers seven areas for assessment:

► trainee assessment
► teaching skills
► the educational process
► teaching resources
► setting objectives
► attitudes
► trainers' learning needs.

These scales are comprehensive and challenging. They provide a useful resource for trainers to consider (*see* Appendix to this chapter for details).

Trainer assessment marking schedule

This is a schedule used by visiting teams in some deaneries. It is reproduced in the Appendix to Chapter 7. The messages it seems to contain for trainers are:

A Trainers should have a philosophy of training (why do you do it?).
B Trainers should have a structural system of some sort.
C Trainers need appropriate resources (time, space, equipment, patients, books).
D Trainers should be part of a training practice that shares the same philosophy.
E Trainers should be part of a quality-orientated practice.
F Trainers should be good role models.

Summary comments

Although the statutory approval system should ensure a minimum quality of training practice, in many cases this process happens once every three years only. The process of improving the quality of training is progressive and some of these tools can encourage this development.

In the assessment of registrars, many trainers feel that the formative assessment process has been eclipsed by summative assessment. The educational cycle doesn't pedal well if it is imbalanced. Trainers need to try and ensure that the summative assessment processes do not dominate the training year. One method of doing this is to harness these processes and use them to achieve educational objectives.

Appendix to Chapter 8

Summative assessment written submission idea framework

This sheet is a one-page summary of the summative assessment process highlighting important issues at the beginning of the year.

The registrar now has to complete a four-part assessment procedure during the year. The assessments are set at *minimal competence* and aim to identify the weakest 3–5% of registrars. The assessment includes:

1 MCQ: can be sat quarterly. It is suggested registrars attempt this after about three months. Registrars are allowed a number of retakes if required. A computerised MCQ program should enable the registrar to judge when he or she is ready.

2 Audit: registrars need to consider getting this off the ground as soon as possible. There are specific, clearly laid out instructions available: follow these and it is impossible to fail! Registrars should expect a tutorial on this quite early on.

3 Video: registrars have to submit a two-hour video for assessment. It is suggested this is a task to start at about the six-month stage of the year. The sooner the registrar starts to familiarise himself or herself with the video the easier this will be.

4 Trainer's report: a lengthy report covering all aspects of general practice. A policy of open assessment invites the registrar's involvement early on.

At first sight this lot can appear daunting – it is not in practice but it is best approached bit by bit starting early on. The regional advisor sends a more detailed booklet to all registrars, so if they don't have one they should ask.

Notes on completing an audit:

- 'Small is beautiful': the best audits use readily identified and fairly small patient samples.
- 'Your idea is better': although ideas can be suggested, the registrar's own idea is usually better.
- 'Two heads are better than one': registrars should not be afraid to ask for help – from anyone! Registrars should get the staff to help wherever possible (i.e. getting notes out, etc.).
- 'The idea framework': this is a list of possible areas for audit that may stimulate the registrar's thoughts:
  - Clinical
    - disease-related (asthma/hypertension/DM)
    - drug-related (lithium/ACEIs/H2RAs/BFZ)
    - investigation-related (MSUs/X-rays)
    - service-related (minor surgery/child health)
    - others (>75 visits/repeat scripts)
  - Admin
    - appointments (numbers/timing/punctuality)
    - visits (re-/areas)
    - sick notes
    - patient call systems
  - Training – tutorials/half-day release/video work
  - Finance – GMS4/private fees
  - Workload – referrals/visits/mileage/appointments/ telephone use
  - Screening – targets/tetanus/flu jabs/practice health policy
  - Personal – journals read/drugs in bags/attitudes/ PGEA
  - Staffing – courses/attitudes/knowledge
  - IT – computer use
  - Prescribing – personal patterns/PACT.
- 'It's a lottery': the Roche prize is awarded in each area annually for the best submitted project. Many people do not bother submitting for it so registrars should consider the option. It is worth about £200.

► 'The audit game': have a go at playing this for 10 minutes with your trainer. It demonstrates how easy it is to design an audit (*see Education for General Practice* (1998) Feb issue).

Notes:

The theory of audit

Some of the terminology of audit is often misunderstood. The following definitions may help.

Audit	The systematic analysis of the quality of medical care, including the procedures used for diagnosis and treatment, the use of resources and the resulting outcome and quality of life for the patient (DOH).
Tracer	The clinical condition under review, i.e. hypertension, asthma.
Criterion	A component of a clinical condition that can be used to measure quality, e.g. BP control for hypertension, PEFR for asthma.
Standard	The qualitative/quantitative expression of criterion. This can either be ideal (100% of all hypertensives will have a BP <140/80) or optimal (60% of all hypertensives will reach the target).
Target	The attainable target, which will vary from audit to audit and place to place.

Critical event audit	The analysis of an event (usually with a suboptimal outcome) to identify areas for possible change.
Protocol	An agreed set of guidelines on optimal practice (either evidence- or consensus-based) against which good practice can be judged.

The RCP suggest a five-point practical approach to audit:

1 Observe practice.
2 Set a standard.
3 Compare observed practice with the standard.
4 Implement change.
5 Observe again to assess the result of the change.

Many practices perform 'pre-audits, which are essentially surveys that allow the current state of play to be assessed. This is really only an accentuated step 1 above.

Many would suggest the audit cycle is really a helix of continuing change – the conventional cycle is shown in Figure A8.1.

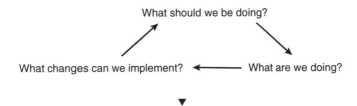

Figure A8.1: The audit cycle.

The Oxford MAAG system in Box A8.1 attempts to classify the quality of practice audits on a structural basis. This may be helpful to assess the level of audit planning in a practice. However, the real value of audit lies in its ability to produce change and increase quality of care. Measuring these is more difficult.

Box A8.1: A classification system for audit

 I   Choose topic
 II   Identify criterion and set standards
 III Data collected, analysed and presented
 IV Discussion among the relevant parties affected
 V   Changes made
 VI Cycle repeated

The audit is then coded:

A five out of six steps present
B codes I and III plus either II or V
C codes I and III
D codes I and intention to audit
E no audit.

Points for discussion: Is this a valid system? What are the strengths/weaknesses of this classification?

Donabedian identified three categories of medical care:

▸ **Structure**: easy to measure (How many PEFR meters have we got?) but limited value.
▸ **Process**: what are we doing? (How many men in the 35–75 year age range have had their BP recorded?) More involved and amenable to change but relies on the assumption that the process affects outcome
▸ **Outcome**: what is the result of our care? (How many asthma admissions have we prevented?) This is the bottom line but is difficult to measure and often a long-term outcome.

Many practices have devised successful process audits that are built on the research evidence that the process does influence outcome.

Issues of medical confidentiality must always be considered in the presentation of audits – anonymise data wherever possible and consider patient, doctor and practice confidentiality (i.e. anonymise all these depending on your audience).

The UKCRA summative assessment written submission marking schedule

Assessors are asked to tick the boxes – all five boxes must be ticked for a clear pass.

Question	Criterion	Criterion present
Why was the audit done?	**Reason for choice** Should be clearly defined and reflected in the title. Should include potential for change	
How was the audit done?	**Criteria chosen** Should be relevant to the subject of the audit. Should be justified	
	Preparation and planning Should show appropriate teamwork and methodology in carrying out the audit.	

Question	*Criterion*	*Criterion present*
	If standards are set they should be appropriate and justified	
What was found?	**Interpretation of data** Should use relevant data to allow conclusions to be drawn	
What next?	**Detailed proposals for change** Should show explicit details of proposed changes	

A satisfactory registrar audit report should include all five criteria to pass.
Please enter your opinion in the box below.

PASS
REFER

If refer, please comment on your reasons.

The design format of the audit submission poses the following questions:

1 What is the title of your audit?
2 Why did you choose it?
3 What criteria have you chosen?
4 Why did you choose them?

5 What preparation and planning did you undertake for your audit project?
6 Have you summarised relevant data?
7 What conclusions do you draw from these?
8 Are the changes you propose as a result of your audit project detailed?
9 Are references included?

MRCGP – statistical terms

> The best way to understand a term is to explain it to someone else
>
> *Anon.*

This list has been used as a pairs exercise to raise awareness of the terms. The trainer and registrar or registrar pairs work down the list explaining alternate terms to each other. The definitions are available (*see* Chapter 10) in statistical books or on the back covers of the evidence-based medicine journal.

Randomised	Bias	Prospective
Retrospective	Double blind	Dropouts
Power	Specificity	Sensitivity
Positive predictive value	Validity	Reliability
Significance	Outcome	Endpoint
Confidence interval	Recruitment	Blind

Generalisability	Observational	Cohort
Longitudinal	Cross-sectional	Interventional
Case-control	Absolute risk reduction (ARR)	Relative risk reduction (RRR)
Standard deviation	Chi-squared test	Mode
Correlation coefficient	Mean	P value
Number needed to treat (NNT)		

MRCGP – critical appraisal

These notes are intended as guidelines both for general reading and to help with the MRCGP examination.

Environment
► Who did the study? Why? Where? Is it relevant to ordinary general practice?

Objectives
► Are they stated? If not can you deduce them?

Design
► What is it?
   – case report
   – case series
   – prospective
   – retrospective

  – cross-sectional
  – intervention/non-intervention
  – longitudinal
  – experimental
  – case-control
  – controlled trial
  – cohort.
► Is it relevant to the study objective stated?
► Could you reproduce it from the details given?

Sample characteristics
► Representative?
► What was the sampling method? Was bias introduced?
  (selection/observer/recall)
► Sample size? Are there statistics to show it is large enough?
► Entry criteria
► Exclusions
► Non-respondents.

Control group characteristics
► How were controls defined?
► What was their source?
► How were they matched/randomised?
► What is the effect of comparable factors?

Quality of measurements/outcomes
► Test characteristics, i.e. validity/sensitivity/specificity/
  reproducibility/reliability
► Blindness?
► Quality control, i.e. calibration exercises/observer
  repeatability tests
► Outcome measures, i.e. defined/valid.

Completeness
► Dropouts/deaths
► Missing data
► Response rates?

Results
- Are they well laid out?
- What about the statistics? (*see* separate list)

Distorting influences
- Contamination, i.e. cases in control group, etc.
- Confounding variables
- Time effects
- Analysis distortions
- Sponsorship?

Conclusions
- Are they justified?

Reference: Foulkes and Fulton (1991).

MRCGP – READER

This is a critical appraisal tool described by Macauley (1994) in the *BJGP*. It can be a simple aide-mémoire when reading a publication.

R Relevance	- to the GP
	- to your own circumstance/patient
	- general awareness
E Education	- would it change your behaviour?
	- would it challenge your beliefs?
A Applicability	- does it seem applicable in your practice?
	- are the results generalisable?
D Discrimination	- what is the quality of the study?
	- what sort of study is it?

	- what about
	   – sample size?
	   – bias?

		– selection?
		– controls?
		– study design?
		– statistics?
		– results?
		– conclusions?
E	Evaluation	▶ reflect on its overall impact/value
R	Reaction	▶ what are you now going to do?

MRCGP – Modular structure 1998

The MRCGP consists of four modules which are marked independently. They can be attempted in any order.

Paper 1	3-hour written paper testing:	application of knowledge critical reading skills awareness of literature data interpretation skills problem solving skills.
Paper 2	3-hour machine marked testing:	knowledge application of knowledge.
Orals	two 20-minute orals testing:	'professional qualities' (attitudes, ethics, etc.)

Consulting skill assessment: a video tape of seven consultations testing consultation skills (a simulated surgery option is available for those that have legitimate reasons for not being able to submit a tape).

Grades

All the modules are marked from A to F, grades E and F are fail grades. Candidates *must* pass all four modules.

The top 25% in each module = merit; 2 × merit = MRCGP with merit; 3–4 × merit = MRCGP with distinction.

- Candidates can resit any module twice (on payment of resit fee).
- Modules can be done in any order.
- Candidates have three years to complete the process.
- Each module is available twice a year – papers 1 and 2 on the same day.
- CPR/CHS certificates necessary on application.

Costs (2000)

- £800 for one attempt at each.
- £200 per module/resit.

End-of-year registrar feedback form

Remember the educational triangle? Well here we are again, only this time it is your turn to look back at the year and evaluate the learning process.

This form allows us to consider elements of the training that perhaps deserve retention in our repertoire and those that need revisiting.

Using any records you have, and considering the *full range* of training activities you have experienced please give us some constructive feedback.

Consider: ▸ clinical teaching (including minor surgery, consultation skills etc)
▸ management teaching
▸ formative and summative assessment
▸ MRCGP teaching
▸ self-development, etc.

A Try and list up to 10 areas/activities that you felt worked well with any comments you feel may help.

B Try and list up to 10 areas/activities that you felt we could improve or add to the year with any comments that may help.

Thank you. Please return this form to the trainer.

The visiting team trainer assessment form

Trainer Assessment Marking Schedule

VISITOR .... TRAINER .... DATE ....

	Poor						Good	
	0	1	2	3	4	5	6	7

The trainer and teaching practice

1 How well has the trainer prepared for the teaching role and to what extent are they keeping up this learning activity?

2 How adequate are the trainer's overall aims?

3 How thorough is the initial assessment of the registrar and the subsequent monitoring?

4 How wide a range of educational method does the trainer employ?

5 How well does the trainer plan and practise protected teaching time?

6 How well is the range of GP topics covered?

7 How well do relationships in the practice combine to produce a good learning environment?

8 How easily can the records be used for teaching?

9 To what extent will the registrar find relevant material in the practice library?

	Poor						Good	
	0	1	2	3	4	5	6	7

10 To what extent does the practice undertake audit and involve the registrar in the evaluation of patient care?   TOTAL/70

Personal attributes of the trainer
1 Energy and enthusiasm
2 Sensitivity and self-awareness
3 Resilience
4 Flexibility

                                                        TOTAL/28

                                         GRAND TOTAL/98

(Teaching skills contribute 42%
Teaching practice features contribute 28%
Personal qualities contribute 30%)

Regional registrar feedback form

CONFIDENTIAL
REGISTRAR ASSESSMENT FORM
Questionnaire for completion by GP trainer at
3, 6 and 11 months (*asterisked questions for
11-month assessment only)

1   Name ....

2   Year graduated ....

3   Address ....

4   Name of trainer ....

5   Structure of VTS: were you on an arranged
    VTS scheme? ....YES/NO

6   *Did you want to do one of the following jobs but
    were unable to find a place to do so:
    Paediatrics   YES/NO
    Obstetrics/Gynaecology   YES/NO

7   *Did you do an introductory general practice
    attachment as part of your vocational training
    scheme (i.e. a period working as a registrar in
    general practice prior to your hospital posts)?
                                             YES/NO

8   *Were you with:
    One practice for 3 months initial and 9 months
    end
    One practice for 12 months
    Two practices for 6 months in each
    Other, please specify ....

9 *Which of these options do you feel is more beneficial for training?
One practice for 3 months initial and 9 months end
One practice for 12 months
Two practices for 6 months in each
Other, please specify ....

10 *During your hospital posts were you able to attend a half-day release course?
Always ( )
Often ( )
Sometimes ( )
Never ( )

11 *Is your half-day release course worth attending?
Always ( )
Often ( )
Sometimes ( )
Never ( )

12 Are you able to attend regional study days if you wish?
Always ( )
Often ( )
Sometimes ( )
Never ( )

13 What is your rota?
1 in 2   1 in 3   1 in 4   1 in 5 or more
Part of cooperative   YES/NO

14 Do you have a set night on-call? If so which night? ....

15 Is the on-call commitment the same as or less than your trainers? ....

16 Do you feel you are working as an extra partner
   rather than a registrar?
   Always ( )
   Often ( )
   Sometimes ( )
   Never ( )

17 Do you feel you work harder than your trainer?
   Always ( )
   Often ( )
   Sometimes ( )
   Never ( )

18 Do you have cover for your surgeries from the
   other partners?
   Always ( )
   Often ( )
   Sometimes ( )
   Never ( )

19 Do you have cover for your night duties from the
   other partners?
   Always ( )
   Often ( )
   Sometimes ( )
   Never ( )

20 Do you feel exploited?
   Always ( )
   Often ( )
   Sometimes ( )
   Never ( )

Comments ....

21 Do you have adequate time for reading?

YES/NO

22 Are the library facilities adequate?   YES/NO

23 How much time does the trainer or other partners spend per week with you on undisturbed teaching (on average)?
Less than 1 hour ( )
1–2 hours ( )
2–3 hours ( )
More than 3 hours ( )

24 How much undisturbed teaching do you feel you need?
Less than 1 hour ( )
1–2 hours ( )
2–3 hours ( )
More than 3 hours ( )

25 Do you have in the practice:

Registrar sitting in on trainer surgery	YES/NO
Trainer sitting in on registrar surgery	YES/NO
Joint home visits	YES/NO
Topic teaching	YES/NO
Random and problem case analysis	YES/NO
Clinical case presentation	YES/NO
Video recording of consultations	YES/NO
Consultation skill analysis	YES/NO
Opportunities to do a project	YES/NO

26 Are there occasions when you cannot attend the day release course due to practice commitments?
Always ( )
Often ( )
Sometimes ( )
Never ( )

27 Do you have to do an evening surgery after the half-day release course?
Always ( )
Often ( )
Sometimes ( )
Never ( )

28 Have you seen an age/sex register *in use* at the practice?   YES/NO

29 Have you seen audit *being used* in the practice?   YES/NO

30 Do you feel your trainer is in a position to assess your:
Knowledge ( )
Clinical skills ( )
Attitudes to patients ( )
Attitudes to staff ( )

31 *How much did your time in practice increase your knowledge concerning the following:

	Very little		A great deal		
	1	2	3	4	5
Practice management					
Practice finance					
Organisation of practice staff					

32 *With respect to general practice in particular how much did your time in practice increase:

	Very little		A great deal		
	1	2	3	4	5
Your clinical knowledge					
Your clinical skills					
Your confidence					

33 Have you signed a contract? YES/NO

34 Have you had help with allowances? YES/NO

35 Are you provided with a bag and equipment?
   YES/NO

36 *Following your vocational training do you feel that you have gained adequate experience and understanding of the GP tasks given below:

Management of minor illness	YES/NO
Management of GP emergencies	YES/NO
Chronic disease protocols	YES/NO
Antenatal care	YES/NO
Postnatal care	YES/NO
Intrapartum care	YES/NO
Family planning	YES/NO
Immunisation	YES/NO
Cervical screening	YES/NO
Preventative care in the elderly	YES/NO
Child health surveillance	YES/NO
Minor surgery	YES/NO

37 Are you enjoying the registrar year? YES/NO

38 Have you any ideas to improve your present training?

39 *Have you any ideas to improve GP training generally?

40 Any other comments?

The Burton trainer rating scales 1–6

Trainer rating scale

This rating scale is modelled on the one used in the Burton Trainers' Workshop. The seven sheets represent seven aspects of the trainer's abilities as a teacher. It can be used in a variety of different circumstances:

- ► by the the trainer as a self–assessment exercise
- ► within a peer group setting to facilitate formative assessment of the trainer
- ► by the trainee to reflect back to the trainer his or her perceived strengths or weaknesses
- ► by a combination of these.

All the sheets, apart from sheets 2 and 4, contain pairs of two opposing statements. Think of these statements as lying at the end of a line containing six points, with number 6 to the left and number 1 to the right. With each pair of statements decide where on that line the trainer in question lies, and write the score in the appropriate box on the recording sheet. The instructions for sheets 2 and 4 are on those sheets.

Sheet 1

Setting objectives

This sheet concerns the clarification and negotiation of hopes, expectations and objectives of both the trainer and the registrar.

---

1 The trainer has clarified his/her objectives for what the registrar is expected to achieve in the training period
    1 2 3 4 5 6   The trainer has no clear idea what the registrar is expected to achieve

2 The trainer has shared those objectives with the trainee
    1 2 3 4 5 6   The registrar does not know what is expected of them

3 The trainer has established what the registrar hopes to achieve in the training period
    1 2 3 4 5 6   The trainer remains unaware of the hopes and expectations of the registrar

4 The trainer has negotiated a training programme based on the objectives of both the registrar and and trainer
    1 2 3 4 5 6   The trainer has either imposed his/her own objectives or accepted the registrar's objectives at face value

---

Sheet 2

Teaching resources

This sheet concerns provision by the trainer and the training practice of the resources for satisfactory training.

Decide on a linear scale of 1–6 how far and how well these resources have been provided so that 6 equals fully provided and 1 equals not provided.

1 A designated, if not exclusive room	1 2 3 4 5 6
2 A medical bag	1 2 3 4 5 6
3 Other diagnostic equipment	1 2 3 4 5 6
4 A well-stocked and up-to-date library	1 2 3 4 5 6
5 Computer facilities	1 2 3 4 5 6
6 Organised, integrated and summarised medical records	1 2 3 4 5 6
7 An introductory guide to the practice and practice systems	1 2 3 4 5 6
8 An annual practice report	1 2 3 4 5 6
9 Video recording and viewing equipment.	1 2 3 4 5 6

Sheet 3

The educational process

This sheet concerns the educational process.

Decide on a linear scale of 1–6 how good the trainer is at organising and executing the teaching process, where 6 equals very good and 1 equals very poor.

1 On the basis of perceived needs the trainer varies the teaching and learning in a flexible manner   1 2 3 4 5 6   The trainer sticks to a rigid educational curriculum and method regardless of the registrar's needs

2 The trainer involves the registrar in planning the content and style of learning activities   1 2 3 4 5 6   The trainer tells the registrar what is to be learnt and how

3 The trainer has experience of, and uses, a range of teaching methods, e.g. discussion, role play, consultation analysis, simulated cases, etc.   1 2 3 4 5 6   The trainer has a narrow range of teaching methods

4 In tutorials the 1 2 3 4 5 6 The trainer
trainer encourages dominates the
the registrar to the tutorial giving
think and talk for the registrar little
him/herself chance to put
an independent view

5 The trainer involves 1 2 3 4 5 6 The trainer fails to
other members of use the members
the practice and of the team to
the extended teach
healthcare team,
in the teaching
process

6 The trainer 1 2 3 4 5 6 The trainer is
encourages a wide reluctant to allow
variety of learning the registrar to
opportunities, leave the practice
e.g. exchange visits, for outside visits
study days, etc.

7 The trainer values 1 2 3 4 5 6 The trainer
the registrar's emphasises the
on-call commitment service element of
as a learning the on-call duties
opportunity

Sheet 4

Teaching skills

This sheet assesses the competence of the trainer to teach or facilitate learning in a range of general practice topics.

Decide on a linear scale of 1–6 how good the trainer is at teaching or facilitating learning in the following topics, where 6 equals very good and 1 equals very poor.

1 Rheumatology and orthopaedics	1	2	3	4	5	6
2 Ophthalmology	1	2	3	4	5	6
3 ENT	1	2	3	4	5	6
4 Children's medicine	1	2	3	4	5	6
5 Child health surveillance	1	2	3	4	5	6
6 General medicine	1	2	3	4	5	6
7 General surgery	1	2	3	4	5	6
8 Dermatology	1	2	3	4	5	6
9 Psychiatry	1	2	3	4	5	6
10 Obstetrics and gynaecology	1	2	3	4	5	6
11 Contraception	1	2	3	4	5	6
12 Minor surgery	1	2	3	4	5	6
13 The consultation	1	2	3	4	5	6
14 Interpersonal relationships	1	2	3	4	5	6
15 Audit	1	2	3	4	5	6
16 Research	1	2	3	4	5	6
17 Business and administration in practice	1	2	3	4	5	6
18 Computers	1	2	3	4	5	6
19 Ethics	1	2	3	4	5	6
20 Prevention and screening	1	2	3	4	5	6

Sheet 5

Registrar assessment

This sheet assesses the abilities of the trainer in assessing the registrar.

Decide on a linear scale of 1–6 how good the trainer is at assessing the registrar, where 6 equals very good and 1 equals very poor.

1	The trainer is enthusiastic about assessing the registrar	1 2 3 4 5 6	The trainer sees assessment as an intrusive and irrelevant chore
2	The trainer is able to provide an individualised, detailed and fair assessment of the registrar's strengths and weaknesses	1 2 3 4 5 6	The trainer provides only superficial and generalised assessment of the registrar
3	The trainer provides assessment of the registrar at regular intervals of no more than three months	1 2 3 4 5 6	The trainer's assessment is irregular or non-existent

4 The trainer uses a   1   2   3   4   5   6   The trainer uses
variety of assessment only limited
techniques – sitting assessment
in, joint surgeries, techniques
video-recording,
patient and staff
feedback rating
scales, etc.

5 The trainer   1   2   3   4   5   6   The trainer makes
documents the few records of any
assessments made assessments made
in a reliable and
consistent manner

6 The trainer takes   1   2   3   4   5   6   The trainer feeds
time to feed back back any
assessments to the assessments to the
registrar in a registrar in an
protected, specified informal
environment unstructured
manner

7 The trainer's   1   2   3   4   5   6   The trainer's
feedback is helpful feedback is
and constructive unhelpful and
destructive

Sheet 6

Attitudes

This sheet assesses the trainer's attitudes which are fundamental in providing a motivating and facilitating environment for the registrar.

1	The trainer is caring and compassionate about the registrar's emotional and intellectual development	1 2 3 4 5 6	The trainer is unconcerned about the registrar's welfare
2	The trainer is conscientious about preparing for tutorials and other learning opportunities for the registrar	1 2 3 4 5 6	The trainer prepares sessions in a slapdash manner
3	The trainer is punctual and keeps to pre-arranged times	1 2 3 4 5 6	The trainer is often late and fails to respect the registrar's time
4	The trainer is interested in, and enthusiastic about the learning process	1 2 3 4 5 6	The trainer is uninterested in teaching and learning

5 The trainer is easily 1 2 3 4 5 6 The trainer is often
   approachable   busy, pre-occupied
   even when busy   and unresponsive to
                                               the registrar's
                                               problems

6 The trainer is   1 2 3 4 5 6 The trainer is
   likeable and has   often brusque,
   good personal   difficult to talk to
   relationships inside   and get on with
   and outside the
   practice

7 The trainer   1 2 3 4 5 6 The trainer
   recognises and   expects the
   values any   registrar to be
   differences in   exactly like
   personality   him/herself
   between him/
   herself and the
   registrar

Sheet 7

Trainer's learning needs

This sheet concerns the trainer's own learning needs and his or her willingness to change and develop.

Decide on a linear scale of 1–6 how good the trainer is at identifying and meeting their own educational needs, where 6 equals very good and 1 equals very poor.

---

1 The trainer is interested in keeping up to date with medical advances and developments

   1 2 3 4 5 6

The trainer shows little interest in his/her own learning and is out of touch with medical advances

2 The trainer reads extensively and has a good grasp of the range of current medical literature.

   1 2 3 4 5 6

The trainer reads little and then only from a narrow range of medical literature

3 The trainer is an active member of the local trainers' workshop

   1 2 3 4 5 6

The trainer either rarely attends, or is an unenthusiastic member of the local workshop

4 The trainer is able 1 2 3 4 5 6 The trainer is unable
to recognise his/her   to recognise his/her
own learning needs   own learning needs
and set appropriate   and takes no steps
learning objectives   to address them

5 The trainer   1 2 3 4 5 6 The trainer has little
periodically seeks   or no interest in
assessment of his/   assessing his/her
her own performance   own performance
from others, e.g.
registrar, partners,
colleagues, patients

Technical aspects of video-taping: what advice can trainers offer on the technical aspects of producing a good quality video tape?

Vorsprung durch Technik (advance through technology)

Ascribed to Hooper

Introduction

Some deaneries have produced guidelines covering the technical aspects of good quality video production. None of us is a Hollywood director but there is a huge variation in the quality of tapes submitted for assessment. How do the best ones do it?

Finance

Essentially you get what you pay for, so buy the best camera you can afford and don't forget a decent TV (remember the one about putting new wine in old skins) – you can have the best camera in the world but on an old black and white 10-inch screen it isn't going to show well!

In our survey, practices financed this from patient donations, local health authority grants (if you don't ask you don't get), GPFH, drug representatives, local support groups (rotary, etc.), the training grant (although £1000–£2000 makes a big hole in this), practice incentive schemes and some even from their own pocket. Remember it is tax deductable and this lightens the load a little.

Suppliers

Trainers use a variety of suppliers. Some deanery GP departments have links with specific suppliers and can recommend them (certainly the West Midlands have). Try borrowing the model you are considering to see if it suits your needs. Look in *Which?* magazine (*see* the IT section in Chapter 11 for the *Which?* site).

Many trainers recommended local suppliers for the benefit of local support. Expect to spend in the region of £600–£1500 (1998 prices).

Features/types

- ▶ General: buy the simplest design that fits your requirements. Many have features you will never use.
- ▶ Size: look for a discreet design, although there is a trade-off here. Small cameras use the smaller tapes, which only last for about 60 minutes. You can buy an expanding cassette so they don't have to be transposed but you are still limited in time. The larger VHS models will still fit discreetly in a room and can run for 3–4 hours. Larger cameras are generally more expensive.
- ▶ Controls: a remote control is essential.

Monitors

Consider a TV/video combined unit, although the quality of the picture must be checked. Certainly buy a TV with a good size screen.

The room

Consider using a dedicated room that is quiet and has the right lighting requirements (see below). Traffic outside, noisy corridors and air conditioning units are real problems. Most trainers recommend a permanent wall bracket, but remember requirements for power sockets and lead runs (remote controls and microphones) when you position this. There were mixed feelings about tripods, with the majority feeling they were intrusive. Try and avoid using batteries as a power source for any purpose – batteries go flat, power companies do not! Check the field of vision the camera will achieve and consider floor markers for chairs to help you stay 'on-screen'. Try and ensure an 'off-screen' area for examinations or fit the lens cap while doing these. If you examine in a separate room consider how you will still record the sound in this room (most doctors continue consulting skills activity during examinations). It is probably best if the registrar's normal consulting room is chosen. A bare room produces echoes so consider a room with wallpaper, carpets and other furniture.

Picture quality and lighting

The best picture comes from an evenly lit room with abundant natural light. Avoid the backlighting effect of windows in the field of vision. If possible have the camera facing away from the window. Some cameras will have a 'backlight compensator' to help cope with this. If you are sufficiently skilled you can use a light meter but not one trainer mentioned this. Consider drawing the curtains if the window is a real problem and have good artificial light. Be careful that these lights illuminate the scene and not the lens or you will simply create the same problem. Most cameras will cope with fairly low light conditions but some have specific low-light capabilities that may suit your requirements. Avoid PC flicker if possible by keeping the PC monitor out of the picture. Include the doctor and the patient in the picture – you will need a wide angle lens facility.

Sound quality

Poor sound quality is a common problem. Start well by using a quiet room on a quiet day. Try and limit background noise; tell the staff not to interrupt (you can always hope). Computer printers create an awful noise on camera and this can be minimised either by turning it off, positioning microphones away from it and placing it on a mat to limit vibration and sound conduction. Desktop remote microphones were highly recommended (Tandy was mentioned as a cheap supplier). The flat variety can be Blu-tacked to the desk to limit movement (try this on the printer as well). Avoid battery microphones – you never notice the battery is flat until after the 'perfect' consultation has just occurred! The microphone should be 3–4 feet from the doctor and patient.

Editing

This can be time-consuming but many trainers feel it is easy when you know how. Ensure you have the right cabling and don't try to be too clever (i.e. fades, etc.). A scart socket on the camera will facilitate editing and improve editing quality. It seems to be easier on combined

TV/video units. Integral screens facilitate editing and standard VHS tapes also make the process smoother. Medical photography departments may be able to help, but remember the confidentiality issues if you are using a local department. Trainers should allow the registrar time to do this.

Process

Brief the staff and consider video-taping a regular session to get everyone used to the idea. Ask them to tell patients that this session will be video-taped when they make the appointment. Keep the consenting procedure out of the consultation room. Have the staff deal with the pre- and post-consultation signatures and get them to chase missed forms. Ensure the correct forms are used and that the GMC guidance procedures are followed (*see* Appendix to this chapter). Consider video-taping at quiet times (half days, Saturdays) and consider lengthening the appointment times as appropriate. Set the camera going at the start of the session and leave it running whenever possible. If you keep turning it off and on, invariably it will be off when you want it on and vice versa. Keep a note of each consultation and particularly 'the good, the bad, the ugly' and the interesting.

Other points to note

Modern cameras can do just about everything except make a cup of tea. Many trainers felt the following points were useful. Buy a camera with an internal clock. Consider one with a slow-play facility to lengthen your tape capacity but remember this may not be suitable for summative assessment or MRCGP use. Most cameras have an autofocus function, which generally works well. However, if the patient and the doctor face each other and the background is more than a few feet away, the camera will focus on the far objective, blurring the doctor and patient. The camera may need to be focused manually in this situation. If you are filming in artificial light look in the manual and consider a 'white balance' adjustment. Always check the quality of the filming (picture and sound) prior to going 'live'.

Advice

If you need help consider:

- techno-wizard partner/registrars/staff
- your supplier
- medical photography department
- course organiser/regional GP department.

Three final points:

- DON'T forget security and insurance (these things walk).
- DON'T forget a supply of tapes and to put one in!
- DON'T forget to switch it on (you may laugh but...).

Notes:

Appendix to Chapter 9

The process of video-recording consultations

Consent forms

The summative assessment consent form can be downloaded from the West Midlands Postgraduate Education website (www.pmde.com). This form fulfils the GMC guidelines but all registrars should ensure they are using the correct form for their area.

The MRCGP consulting skills (video) component consent form can be downloaded from the College website: http://rcgp.org.edu/

GMC guidelines

This page contains the GMC guidelines on the video-recording of consultations.

General Medical Council
Video-recording of consultations between doctors and patients and of other medical procedures for the purposes of training and assessment.

Guidance

1 Medical procedures involving patients may be recorded on video tape, audio tape or on film for the purposes of assessment or training only where the patient has given free and informed consent. Where the recording involves a consultation between doctor and patient or any other procedure from which the patient may be identified, and if the recording may cause the patient embarrassment or other distress, doctors are responsible for ensuring the following:

In advance of the recording:

(a) The patient understands the purpose for which the recording would be used, who would be allowed to see it, including the names of the people if known, whether copies would be made and how long the recording would be kept.

(b) The patient understands that a refusal to consent to recording will not affect the quality of care being offered.

(c) The patient is given time to consider a consent form and explanatory material that sets out the necessary information in a way which the patient can understand (translation should be provided where necessary).

(d) The consent form is neutrally worded, in order not to imply that consent is expected.

(e) Where patients are unable to give consent because they suffer from a mental disability, or for any other reason, consent must be sought from a close relative or carer. In the case of children who lack the understanding to consent on their own behalf, the consent of a parent or guardian must be obtained. The person giving consent must understand the rights set out above and below.

During the recording:

(f) The recording must be stopped immediately if the patient requests or if, in the doctor's opinion, recording is reducing the benefit that the patient might derive from the consultation.

After the recording:

(g) The patient is invited after the recording to consider whether to vary or withdraw the consent to use the recording.

(h) Where, following a recording, the patient withdraws or fails to confirm consent, the recording must be erased as soon as possible.

(i)   The recording is used only for the purposes for which the patient's consent was obtained.

(j)   The recording is stored with the security required for all confidential medical records.

(k)   The recording is erased in accordance with the patient's instructions.

These conditions also apply to any copies of a video-recording.

2   Where a video-recording is or may be shown to people other than the healthcare team immediately responsible for the care of the patient at the place where the recording is made the following additional safeguards should be applied:

(a)   The patient must understand that the recording may be shown to people with no responsibility for the patient's healthcare.

(b)   The patient must be offered the opportunity to view the recording, in the form in which it is intended to be shown, before the recording is used, and have the right to withdraw consent to use the recording at that stage.

3   Where it is proposed to make a recording from which the patient cannot be identified, it is sufficient for the doctor to give the patient an oral explanation of the purpose of the proposed recording and to seek the patient's consent, which should be recorded in the notes. No recording should be made contrary to the patient's wishes, and no pressure should be placed on a patient to consent. In exceptional circumstances, where on recording of a procedure that has been planned, an unexpected development during the procedure makes a recording highly desirable on educational grounds, a recording may be made without consent if the patient's consent cannot be sought (for example because of anaesthesia). In such circumstances the patient's consent must be obtained before use is made of the recording.

CHAPTER 10

Resources: what information technology and reference sources are trainers using?

Where shall I find all the time to do this non-reading?

Krauss

Introduction

Many trainers are hoarders – they produce collections of references, pictures, slides, tapes and props of all sorts. These are very individual collections and are sometimes used and sometimes not. Some trainers dislike this approach. This chapter offers suggestions that may be useful. It will often be ideal for the registrar to search for his or her own references, but life is life, people are people and these resources may be more pragmatic at times.

Most of the items in this list of references have proved useful over a number of years. Some will date but usually they relate to the principles or the process in that area, or are considered important or 'seminal' work.

We believe all the references and resources are described in sufficient detail for trainers to find or order them. Some items may be out of publication – established trainers can be a useful source of these.

References – for registrars

This list includes references trainers have found useful in teaching registrars. It is not all-inclusive and space is left in each section for additions. In practice, most trainers have easy access to the *BMJ* and *BJGP* and the majority of references are not surprisingly from these journals. In most instances there should be enough detail to find the reference.

*Papers that particularly lend themselves to a tutorial with a critical appraisal element.

Asthma
- BTS guidelines (revised 1997)   *Thorax* (1993) March.
- Diagnosis   *BMJ* Editorial (1997) 5 July.

Cardiology
- *Use of ECG in diagnosis of heart failure   *BMJ* (1996) Jan.
- SOLVD   *NEJM* (1992) **327**: 685–91.
- CONSENSUS II   *NEJM* (1992) **327**: 678–84.
- SHEP   *JAMA* (1991) **265**: 3255–64.
- SAVE   *NEJM* (1992) **327**: 669–77.
- Fibrinolysis   *Lancet* (1994) **343**: 311–22.
- STOP   *Lancet* (1991) **338**: 1281–5.
- Antiplatelet trialist collaboration   *BMJ* (1988) **296**: 320–1.
  BMJ (1994) **308**: 81–106.
- OXCHECK   *BMJ* (1994).
- Aspirin side effects   *BMJ* (1995) Jan.
- Angina – consensus guidelines   *BMJ* (1996) 30 Mar.
- AF and stroke – review   *Archives of Internal Medicine* (1994) July.

Cholesterol

- Scandinavian Simvastatin survival study — *Lancet* (1994) Nov.
- CARE — *NEJM* (1996).
- West of Scotland coronary prevention study — *BMJ* (1997) **315**: 7122.

Complementary medicine

- Acupuncture review — *Update* (1997) 21 May.
- A measure of success — *BJGP* (1997) Jan.

Consultation and patient care

- Improving skills — *BJGP* (1996) July.
- The patient-centred clinical method — *Family Practice* (1986) **3**: 24–30.
- What do patients think? — *BJGP* (1996) Sep.
- The elderly and communication problems — *Ageing and Society* (1991) **11**: 127–48.
- Patients' role in decision making — *Annals of Internal Medicine* (1980) **93**: 718–22.
- Heartsink patients — *BMJ* (1988) **297**: 20–7.
- The difficult doctor/patient relationship: somatisation, personality and psychopathology — *Journal of Clinical Epidemiology* (1994) **47**(6): 647–57.
- Empathy: an essential skill for understanding the physician/patient relationship in clinical practice — *Family Medicine* (1993) **25**(4): 245–8.
- Doctor/patient relationship: Toronto consensus (good reference section in this paper) — *BMJ* (1991) **303**: 1385–7.

▶ Patients with unexplained and vexing medical complaints

Journal of General Internal Medicine (1988) **3**: 177–90.

Counselling
▶ Counselling in GP　　　　*BJGP* (1994) **44**: 194–5.

Critical reading
▶ How to read a paper　　　*BMJ* series from July 1997.
▶ Critical appraisal of published research　　*BMJ* (1991) **302**: 1136–40.

Diabetes
▶ DCCT　　　　　　　　*NEJM* (1993) **329**: 977–86.
▶ Shared care　　　　　　*BMJ* Editorial (1995) **310**: 142–3.

Evidence-based medicine
▶ Socratic dissent　　　　*BMJ* (1995) **310**: 1126–7.
▶ EBM – an approach to clinical problem solving　　*BMJ* (1995) **310**: 1122–6.
▶ Series in *BMJ*　　　　*BMJ* (1998) **317** July to Aug.

Epidemiology/public health
▶ Income inequality and mortality　　　*BMJ* (1996) series Apr.
▶ Poverty and social influences on health　　*BMJ* (1997) series Feb.
▶ Inner cities (Black report)　　　RCGP Occasional paper.

Ethics
▶ Four principles plus scope　　　*BMJ* (1994) 16 July.
▶ Drug representative visits　　　*BMJ* (1996) May.

▶ Ethical aspects of   *BJGP* (1992) **42**: 486.
medical certification
by GPs

GU medicine

▶ Detection of cancer   *BMJ* (1995) **310**: 140–1.
of the prostate

HRT

▶ American nurses study *JAMA* (1996).
▶ Use of HRT   *BJGP* (1995) **45**: 355–8.

Investigations/diagnosis

▶ *Use of the normal   *BMJ* (1996) 18 Aug.
investigation to
reassure
▶ Interpretation of   *BJGP* (1985) **35**: 270–4.
diagnostic data
▶ There's a lot of it about: *BJGP* (1986) **36**: 468–71.
clinical strategies in
family practice
▶ Diagnostic investig- *Canadian Family Physician*
ations in family practice (1989) **35**: Oct.
▶ Problem solving and *Canadian Family Physician*
decision making in (1979) **25**: 1473.
family practice

LBP

▶ Management paradigm *BMJ* Editorial (1996) Nov.
after RCGP guidelines

Management

▶ Managing change in   *BMJ* (1992) **304**: 231–4.
GP: a step-by-step
guide
▶ Practice nurses and   *BMJ* (1995) Mar.
minor illness

- ► Computers in the consulting room   *BJGP* (1994) Aug.
- ► Night cover in general practice   *BMJ* (1997) Jan.
- ► Opportunity for choice   DoH.
- ► Delivering the future   DoH.
- ► Better living, better life   DoH.
- ► Core services   GMSC.
- ► Practice nurse workload   *BJGP* (1995) **45**: 415–18.

Maternity

- ► Traditional/'New' antenatal care   *BMJ* (1996) Mar.
- ► Changing childbirth   Expert Maternity Group, HMSO/DoH.

Paediatrics

- ► Recognising meningococcal disease in primary care   *BMJ* (1998) **316**: 276–9.
- ► Listen to parents: they know best   *BMJ* (1996) **313**: 954–5.
- ► *What worries parents when their pre-school children are acutely ill and why?   *BMJ* (1996) **313**: 983–6.
- ► Parents difficulties and information needs in coping with acute illness in pre-school children   *BMJ* (1996) **313**: 987–90.
- ► *Otitis media   *BMJ* (1997) **314**: 1526–9.

Prescribing

- ► The doctor's bag   DTB (1995) **33**: 19 Jan.
- ► Towards more rational prescribing in GP   Audit commission report. *BMJ* Comment (1994) **308**: 731.

Professional development

- Life, your career and the pursuit of happiness — *BMJ* Classified (1997) **25** Oct: 2.
- Stress in GP — *BMJ* (1994) **b**: 1261–3.
- Attitudes to medical care: the organisation of work and stress amongst GPs — *BJGP* (1992) **42**(358): 181–5.

Psychiatry/neurology

- Anxiety — *BMJ* (1995) **309**: 321.
- How to perform a rapid neurological examination — *Update* (1997) 1 Oct.
- Unrecognised psychiatric illness in primary care — *BJGP* (1996) Jun.
- Making shared care work — RCP/RCGP report 1995.
- Dizziness – assessment in primary care — *BMJ* (1996) 28 Sep.
- Grief — *BJGP* (1997) July/Aug.
- Defeat depression — RCPsych/RCGP.
- Defeat depression — *BJGP* Editorial (1995) **45**: 170.
- Systematic approach to brief psychotherapy in primary care settings — *Journal of Family Practice* (1978) 7(6): 1137–42.

Referrals

- The gatekeeper and the wizard — *BMJ* (1989) **298**: 172–4.
- The gatekeeper and the wizard revisited — *BMJ* (1992) **304**: 969–71.

Screening

- >75 screening — *BJGP* (1997) Jan.

▶ Screening can damage your health	*BMJ* Editorial (1997) Feb.

Substance abuse

▶ Use of nicotine patches to stop smoking	*Lancet* (1987) July.
▶ Methadone use	*BJGP* Editorial (1995) Sep.

Teenagers

▶ Sex and risk taking	*BMJ* (1993) **307**: 25.

Terminal care

▶ I desperately needed to see my son	*BMJ* (1991) **302**: 356.
▶ An open letter to my surgeon	*BMJ* (1992) **305**: 4 July.

Some of the papers are from more obscure journals. Copies of these can either be obtained from the local postgraduate centre librarian or found on Medline (*see* below).

References – for trainers

This list includes references trainers have found useful in developing their own teaching skills.

▶ Learning by reflection	Al-Sheri, *Education for General Practice* (1995) **7**: 237–48.
▶ The emotional diary: a framework for reflective learning	Howard, *Education for General Practice* (1997) **8**: 288–91.
▶ Personal construct analysis	Dunn, *Education for General Practice* (1993) **2**: 121–5.
▶ Role modelling: a case study in GP	Lublin, *Medical Education* (1992) **26**: 116–22.
▶ The continuum of problem based learning	Harden *et al.*, *Medical Teacher* (1998) **20**: 317.

▶ Motivation to learn	Miller *et al.*, *BJGP* (1998) Jul: 1430.
▶ Independent learning among GP trainees: an initial survey	Bligh, *Medical Education* (1992) **26**: 497–50.
▶ How we teach key aspects of GP	Strasser, *Medical Teacher* (1991) **1**: 93.
▶ Avoiding the myths: a pre-requisite for teaching ethics	Seedhouse, *Education for General Practice* (1992) **3**: 117–24.
▶ Assessment of trainer performance in RCA	Turner *et al.*, *Education for General Practice* (1998) **9**: 199–202.
▶ Assessment of the tutorial	Ruscoe, *Education for General Practice* (1994) **5**: 260–8.
▶ Pathologies of 1:1 teaching	Pitts, *Education for General Practice* (1996) **7**: 118–22.
▶ The S-SDRLS: a short questionnaire about self-directed learning	Bligh, *Education for General Practice* (1993) **4**: 121–5.

All of these articles come from three postgraduate medical education journals. Most trainers found *Education for General Practice* (the 'Green Journal') the most relevant. Details of all three are given below.

▶ *Education for General Practice* is available from Radcliffe Medical Press.
▶ *Medical Education* is available from Blackwell Scientific.
▶ *Medical Teacher* is available from Carfax Publishing Ltd, Abingdon OX14 3UE; web site: http://www.carfax.co.uk.

Other resources

- *If Only I Had the Time*: a joint ICI/RCGP (1989) publication. A distance learning package on time management. The resource book with this package is very good. This was published about 10 years ago and may be difficult to find – some more established trainers may have copies.
- *Promoting Child Health*: this is a manual and two videos covering child health surveillance available from Radcliffe Medical Press. It is useful to cover child health examination issues.
- *Prostate Problems*: GP trainer pack: available from the MSD foundation covering BPH and cancer of the prostate with a variety of literature.
- *Migraine Workshop*: a literature-based module to cover migraine available from Medicom UK.
- *Moving to Audit*: a sequential scenario package looking at the problems of audit. Available from the University of Dundee or from existing trainers.
- *Primary Care Mental Health Toolkit*: a selection of material designed to help educate the PHCT in mental health issues. Produced by the RCGP.
- *3 Minute Neurological Examination*: a video available from Zeneca demonstrating a very GP-orientated neurological examination.
- *Say the Right Thing*: a video from BBC for Business BBC Worldwide Ltd (1995) on assertive language.
- *Straight Talking: the art of assertiveness*: a video from Video Arts (1991) on assertiveness.

Audio cassettes

Medikasset, drug companies and more recently Medical Monitor produce audio cassettes on various subjects. These can be useful prompts for registrars and can be a good way to use the 'marginal time' lost in travelling – listen while you drive!

CD-ROM

An increasing amount of material is becoming available using this medium. Bayer produces useful examples on STDs and chest infections.

Anatomical models

Commercial models for joint injection of the shoulder, knee and wrist are expensive to buy but can be borrowed from Ciba-Geigy via the local representative.

Some practices own or borrow resuscitation dummies (candidates for the MRCGP must submit a CPR competency certificate from an accredited CPR trainer). In the West Midlands, undergraduate training practices linked to the University of Birmingham are now equipped with a large range of anatomical models. These models are used to teach pelvic examinations, ophthalmoscopy, suturing and cardiopulmonary resuscitation.

Films

The following films have some potential for use in training (many of these are taken from the UBC Residents handbook):

- *Dad* – a son connecting with a dying father
- *Long day's journey into night* – alcoholism
- *One flew over the cuckoo's nest* – mental illness
- *The best little girl in town* – anorexia
- *Nothing in common* – divorce and families
- *Whose life is it anyway* – paraplegia/assisted suicide
- *A duet for one* – a musician with MS.

Other

This is another potentially endless list that challenges trainers to be visionary in their use of resources:

- Using topical newspaper cuttings.

- ▶ The Dundee 'CASE' booklets, which show the GP management spectrum and have excellent 'key' point sections. Available from Dundee University.
- ▶ The use of 'prompt cards' for certain subject areas. Previously available from Modern Medicine, Franks Hall, Horton Kirby, Kent. Copies may only be available from fellow trainers now.
- ▶ Using the *Nature of Family Practice* by Fabb *et al.* Series which contains patient scenarios grouped by problem area with accompanying question prompts. Available from Health Science Press.
- ▶ Basing a discussion on one of the RCGP Occasional papers or reports. These are listed in the *BJGP*.
- ▶ CHECK programme. This is a series of booklets to work through individually with a question/answer and clinical case format. They are available from the RACGP and are a comprehensive and useful series of booklets.

Summary comments

A bad workman blames his tools

Anon.

If the quotation is true then perhaps the good workman is equally appreciative of his tools. Despite this, trainers need to keep an eye open for a number of pitfalls: the favourite tool doesn't do every job, i.e. be careful that the teaching is learner-centred and not simply for the trainer's amusement. Don't use a hammer for every job or as one trainer put it 'don't go into auto-pilot'. Trainers need to reflect on the appropriateness and usefulness of their teaching methods and beware of trotting out last years 'lesson'. However, good workmen employ a range of tools for a range of tasks and this section describes some of the resources trainers use.

CHAPTER 11

The written word: what books do trainers recommend? What other sources of information do trainers use?

Some books are undeservedly forgotten: none are undeservedly remembered

Auden

Introduction

The doubling time of total available knowledge is an interesting concept. At the turn of the 20th century it probably took 50 years for the total of all world knowledge to double. By the 1950s it was about five years, in 1980 about three months, and now it is estimated in days. How long before it is in hours, minutes or even seconds? With this rate of progression it is difficult to see how the printed word can keep up! Doctors need to be able to access salient information and to work with a 'playable hand' of this data. Future generations will have to learn to cope with this problem, perhaps without books – but we are not there yet. This chapter describes the books trainers recommend. The details listed for each book are sometimes not as comprehensive as we would have desired. However, there should be enough detail to order or find the book.

General advice

Patterns of reading habits vary enormously. Some doctors seem to read very little but remain well informed using other methods. Some doctors read extensively and seem relatively uninformed. Others seem to acquire a vast data of knowledge but possess little wisdom. Some stand out as both knowledgeable and wise.

Many registrars have developed poor reading habits. They seem to fall into a number of patterns:

▶ *All or nothing reading*: the registrar thinks he or she should read everything. Anyone who seriously tries this will end up reading nothing. Some seem to start at the nothing level.

▶ *Biblical reading*: the registrar is determined to find *a* book that will answer all their worries. This can work at the undergraduate medicine level but not in general practice.

▶ *Binge reading*: the registrar reads in patches but has no regular habit and usually resents the process, i.e. it is done for tutorial preparation, exams or presentations only.

▶ *Comfort reading*: the registrar tends to read about areas they already know and avoids other areas providing a false sense of reassurance and security.

The trainer can facilitate the evolution of a good reading habit in many ways. It is generally accepted that the retention of knowledge from reading is maximised by spending at least an equal (if not greater) time deliberately recalling/rehearsing new learning as is spent actually reading. The role modelling approach is helpful by demonstrating a positive attitude to reading. Pragmatic advice can be given and the Appendix to this chapter contains an example of an advice sheet for registrars. The concepts of reflective learning (*see* Chapter 3) can be used to focus the registrar to read relevant areas related to their experience. Finally the trainer can suggest (or even directly supply) the book to be read.

Books

The list of books in Table 11.1 was considered recommended reading by trainers. The figure in the first column indicates the percentage of trainers who mentioned each book. Each trainer was asked to suggest up to six books. The list contains short notes at the end of each grouping. The list can be used to identify recommended books in specific areas.

Table 11.1: Recommended reading

Subject area/title	Author	Identification
Consultation		
29% Inner Consultation	Neighbour	Kluwer Press (ISBN 0746200404)
24% The Consultation: an approach to learning and teaching	Pendleton & Schofield	Oxford GP Series No 6, (ISBN 0192613499)
11% The Doctor's Communication Handbook (2e)	Tate	Radcliffe Medical Press (ISBN 1857752562)
9% The Doctor, His Patient and the Illness	Balint	Pitman Medical (ISBN 0443036152)
5% Doctors Talking to Patients	Byrne & Long	HMSO (ISBN 850840929)
3% Games People Play	Berne	Penguin Books
2% Teaching Interpersonal Skills	Burnard	Chapman and Hall (ISBN 0412345900)
1% The Doctor–Patient Relationship	Freeling & Browne	Churchill Livingstone (ISBN 0443023751)
1% Six Minutes for the Patient	Balint & Norell	Tavistock Press (ISBN 422742708)
1% Relating to the Relatives: breaking bad news, communication and support	Brewin & Sparshott	Radcliffe Medical Press (ISBN 1857750810)
1% The 15 Minute Hour: applied psychotherapy for the primary care physician	Stuart *et al.*	Praegar Press (ISBN 0275920224)

Table 11.1: Continued

Subject area/title	Author	Identification
Consultation		
1% Skills for Communicating with Patients	Silverman *et al.*	Radcliffe Medical Press (ISBN 1857751892)
1% Teaching and Learning Communication Skills in Medicine	Silverman *et al.*	Radcliffe Medical Press (ISBN 1857752732)
1% Individual Psychotherapy and the Science of Psychodynamics	Malan	Butterworth-Heinemann (ISBN 075062387X)
1% The Doctor, the Patient and the Group	Balint	Routledge (ISBN 0415080533)
1% How to Break Bad News	Buckman	Johns Hopkins University
1% Talking Sense	Asher	Pitman Press
1% Talking with Patients	Myerscough & Ford	Oxford Medical Publications (ISBN 0192616218)
1% The Official Doctor/ Patient Handbook		Duckworth

Notes: the front runners here are self-evident. Apart from these, Tate's The *Doctor's Communication Handbook* gives a relatively brief overview for registrars. At the other extreme Silverman *et al.*'s books provide a detailed breakdown of the component elements of consultation skills that can be very useful in teaching. An awareness of the others is probably wise (at least for anyone sitting the MRCGP) but very few registrars will have the time to read them.

Subject area/title	Author	Identification
Clinical medicine		
11% ABC series in general	Various	BMA Books
10% Oxford Medical Textbook	Weatherall	Oxford University Press (ISBN 0192627066 (vol. 1)) (ISBN 0192627074 (vol. 2)) (ISBN 0192627082 (vol. 3))
4% A Textbook for Family Medicine	McWhinney	Pitman Press (ISBN 0272798193)
3% Treatment and Prognosis in General Practice	Drury	Heinemann
3% Towards Earlier Diagnosis in Primary Care	Hodgkin	Churchill Livingstone (ISBN 780443016856)
3% Guide to the Guidelines (3e)	Smith	Radcliffe Medical Press (ISBN 1857752864)

Table 11.1: Continued

Subject area/title	Author	Identification
Clinical medicine		
2% Oxford Handbook of Clinical Specialities	Collier *et al.*	Oxford University Press (ISBN 0192621157)
2% Medicine International series	Oxford	Medicine (International) Ltd
1% Practical General Practice	Polmear & Khot	Butterworth (ISBN 0750608676)
1% Merck Manual	Berkov	Merck Research Laboratory (ISBN 091910875)
1% Davidson's Principles and Practice of Medicine	McCleod	Churchill Livingstone (ISBN 0443011842)
1% Clinical Method	Fraser	Butterworth Heinemann (ISBN 075061448X)
1% Clinical Medicine	Kumar & Clarke	Ballière Tindall (ISBN 0702011371)

Notes: these books divide into the traditional medical tomes and those with a primary care inclination. The latter group seem to have more relevance for day-to-day use, although most practice libraries will contain a larger text for reference. Many of these books are now available on CD-ROM (the Merck Manual certainly is). These books date rapidly and can be expensive. Perhaps the rolling Medicine International series is a good way of tackling these problems.

General practice – general

5% Doctors' Dilemmas and Decisions	Essex	BMA Books (ISBN 0727908596)
3% Hot Topics in GP	Starey	Oxford BIOS Scientific Publications (ISBN 1859962106)
2% The Mystery of GP	Heath	Nuffield Provincial Hospitals Trust (ISBN 0900574933)
1% Clinical Effectiveness in Primary Care	Baker	Radcliffe Medical Press (ISBN 1857751299)
1% Follies and Fallacies in Medicine	Shrebeneck & McCormick	Tarragon Press (ISBN 1870781023)
1% The Art of GP	Morell	Oxford Medical Publications (ISBN 019261990X)

Table 11.1: Continued

Subject area/title	Author	Identification
General practice – general		
1% A Guide to General Practice	Oxford Trainee Group	Blackwell Scientific Press (ISBN 0632000244)
1% A Little Book of Doctors' Rules	Meador	Hanley and Belfin (ISBN 1560530618)

Notes: this list contains a wide range of material: from the practical checklists of the Oxford Trainee Group to the one-line wisdoms of *A Little Book of Doctors' Rules*. Many of them look at the philosophies of care inherent in general practice that will tend to interest the registrar once they feel comfortable with the basics (*see* the Educational needs hierarchy, Chapter 3). Certainly thoughts like 'The roads to unfreedom are many: one of them is marked Health for All' (Shrebeneck 1994) are rarely for the first week of training.

Subject area/title	Author	Identification
Evidence-based medicine		
2% Evidence-based GP	Risdale	Churchill Livingstone (ISBN 0179291611X)
2% Evidence-based Medicine	Sackett	Churchill Livingstone (ISBN 0443056862)
2% How to Read a Paper	Greenhalgh	BMA Books
1% Dilemmas in GP	Warren	Butterworth Heinemann

Notes: for better or/and worse we are in the era of EBM. Registrars need to acquire the skills to use EBM and attitudes to handle the concept. The reference section contains some interesting material in these areas. One registrar described Sackett's book as 'interesting but too dense'. The density of the book referred to its usefulness per unit volume. Many registrars are looking for low-density reading and perhaps this is a reasonable request in the era of knowledge overload. Certainly the other three books here are designed to be practical tools of low-density material. The concept of density particularly challenges the authors of books designed to make us think.

Subject area/title	Author	Identification
Teaching-related		
20% The Inner Apprentice	Neighbour	Kluwer (ISBN 0792389832)
3% Learning GP: a structured approach	Sandars & Baron	Pastest Books (ISBN 090689641X)
2% Educating the Future GP (2e)	McEvoy	Radcliffe Medical Press (ISBN 1857752813)
2% A New Kind of Doctor	Tudor Hart	Merlin Press
2% Postgraduate Tutorials in GP (and follow-up book)	Warren	Butterworth Heinemann (ISBN 075062552X)
2% A GP Trainer's Handbook	Hall	Blackwell Scientific
2% A GP Training Handbook	Oxford GP Group	Blackwell Scientific (ISBN 0632010819)

Table 11.1: Continued

Subject area/title	Author	Identification
Teaching-related		
1% Once Upon a Group	Kindred	Published at 20 Dover Street, Southwell, Nottingham
1% Aids to GP	Mead	Churchill Livingstone (ISBN 0443036950)
1% Tutorials in GP	Mead	Pitman Press (ISBN 027279709X)
1% The Nature of Family Practice	Fabb & Marshall	MTP Press (ISBN 0852007264)
1% The Trainer's Companion to GP	Rosen	No other details available
1% Self-directed Learning: a guide for teachers and learners	Knowles	Association Press/Follett (ISBN 0696811169)
1% I'm OK, You're OK	Harris	Pan Books
1% Professional Education for General Practice	Havelock *et al.*	Oxford GP Series No 21 (ISBN 0192626078)
1% Assertiveness at Work	Stubbs	Pan Business/ Management
1% Needs to Know: a guide to needs assessment in primary care	Harris	No other details found
1% Introduction to Neurolinguistic Programming	O'Connor	Aquarian Press
1% Teach Yourself Body Language	Wainwright	Hodder and Stoughton
1% Reflective Practice in Nursing	Palmer	Blackwell Scientific Press (ISBN 0632035978)
1% Primary Care Rheumatology distance learning pack	Bolt	No other details found

Notes: this grouping contains a wide range of material. Mead, Warren and Saunders offer tutorial guidance tools (Warren with knowledge details, the others more structural in nature). Fabb and Marshall's publication includes clinical scenarios covering just about every area you can think of (and a few you can't) with accompanying questions. Many of the other books cover teaching philosophies (Neighbour, Havelock, McEvoy), specific techniques (McEvoy, Hall and many reflected in the titles) or particular areas (in the titles).

Table 11.1: Continued

Subject area/title	Author	Identification
Management		
9% The 'Making Sense of' series (red book, audit, new contract, primary care-led NHS, computers, general practice, partnerships, prescribing, cost rent scheme, the law and general practice, managing change, personnel management, pensions and retirement, complaints procedure)	Various	Radcliffe Medical Press
2% Running a Practice	Jones *et al.*	Croom Helm (ISBN 0856645478)
2% Hired, Fired, or Sick and Tired	Macdonald	Brealey (ISBN 1857881060)
1% Disease Data Book	Fry	Kluwer (ISBN 0852009224)
1% The One Minute Manager	Blanchard	Morrow (ISBN 0688014291)
1% UK Health Care: the facts	Fry	Kluwer (ISBN 0792388666)
1% Motivation and Personality	Maslow	Harper
1% If Only I Had the Time	ICI/RCGP	(ISBN 1871749158)

Notes: most registrars will realise the need for some management learning, but this realisation is often late in the year and the area covered superficially. The profusion of the 'Making sense' series is a daunting prospect for registrars. The smaller books are certainly more 'reader-friendly' at the start of the year. The other more specialised books are described in Chapter 7.

Audit		
2% Medical Audit and GP	Marinker	BMA Books (ISBN 0727902954)
1% Audit in Action		No other details found

Notes: fewer than 10% of trainers mentioned a book on audit. There are quite a number of these books and in view of the statutory nature of the current summative assessment audit, registrars need access to some knowledge source. Perhaps there is a market here for a book – perhaps 'Concise audit'.

Table 11.1: Continued

Subject area/title	Author	Identification
Ethics		
1% Medical Ethics		BMA Books
1% Medicine, Patients and the Law	Brazier	Penguin (ISBN 0140225579)

Notes: many of the books listed in other groupings contain considerable ethical components. The reference section also contains some interesting resources in this area.

Examinations		
9% Notes for the MRCGP	Palmar	Blackwell Scientific
5% MRCGP Study Book	Sandars	Pastest Books (new version on the modular format ISBN 0906896649)
1% MRCGP Examination: a guide for candidates and teachers	Moore	RCGP Books
1% Pass Summative Assessment and the MRCGP	Lindsay	Saunders (ISBN 07020221946)

Notes: registrars are often motivated by the exam process – whether trainers like it or not. Trainers can use this motivation to enhance learning, but to achieve this need a knowledge of the exam process and resources that mimic this process, i.e. MEQ questions in certain areas, oral type questions to cover certain attitudes, etc. These books can help trainers achieve these aims.

Women's health		
8% The Pill	Guillebaud	Oxford University Press (ISBN 0192861263)
(also *Contraception: your questions answered,* by the same author, Churchill Livingstone (ISBN 0443037019)		
7% Women's Problems in GP	McPherson & Anderson	Oxford GP Series No 4 (ISBN 0192615718)
2% Notes for the DRCOG	Kaye	Churchill Livingstone (ISBN 0443029253)

Notes: this is a relatively short list for an important area. Either these books are definitive (and many trainers would say they currently are) or there is a need for new work.

Table 11.1: Continued

Subject area/title	Author	Identification
Paediatrics/child health		
2% Toddler Taming	Green	Century Hutchison (ISBN 0091772583)
2% Essential Paediatrics	Hull & Johnson	Churchill Livingstone (ISBN 0443047820)
1% The Normal Child	Illingworth	Churchill Livingstone, (ISBN 0 443 01907 X)
1% Abdominal Pain in Children	O'Donnell	Blackwell Scientific Publications, (ISBN 0632014060)
1% The Child Surveillance Handbook (2e)	Hall	Radcliffe Medical Press (ISBN 1870905245)
1% Health For All Children	Hall	Oxford University Press (ISBN 0192626566)
1% Manual of Child Development	Lingam & Harvey	Churchill Livingstone (ISBN 04433037841)

Notes: all registrars should have seen the Hall reports and need knowledge resources to cover normal child development, screening and children's illness. *Toddler Taming* promotes insight into the problems of early child care (particularly for anyone who has not experienced the joys of parenthood).

Dermatology

4% Clinical Dermatology Illustrated	Reeves	Balgowlah AOD Health Science Press (ISBN 0867920106)
4% Wolfe: a colour atlas of dermatology	Levene	(ISBN 0723401748)
2% Colour Atlas of Paediatric Dermatology	Verbor & Morley	No other details found

Notes: every training practice should have a dermatology atlas. Take your pick! Many of these atlases also cover the basic details of diagnosis and treatment.

Minor surgery/anatomy

1% Atlas of Minor Surgery	Cracknell	Churchill Livingstone (ISBN 044305309)
1% Grants Method of Anatomy	Grant	(ISBN 0683003720)

Table 11.1: Continued

Subject area/title	Author	Identification
Minor surgery/anatomy		
1% Joint and Soft Tissue Injection (2e)	Silver	Radcliffe Medical Press (ISBN 1857753410)
1% Practice Tips	Murtagh	McGraw-Hill (ISBN 0074528041)

Notes: teaching minor surgery in the practice is a challenge. An anatomy reference book seems essential, with some kind of visual support material and specific technique advice. These books cover these areas but there are others – the challenge will always be converting knowledge into practical competence.

Mental illness		
1% Sanity, Madness and the Family: families of schizophrenics	Laing	Penguin
1% Grief Counselling and Grief Therapy	Worden	Routledge (ISBN 0415071798)

Notes: this is a short list for a large area. Registars need a reference source for general practice mental health problems but no particular book was mentioned.

Other clinical areas		
7% The BNF		BMA/British Pharmaceutical Society HMSO (ISBN 0853693935)
3% Emergencies in GP	Mould	MTP Press (ISBN 0867920262)
2% The Eye in Clinical Practice	Frith	Blackwell Scientific (ISBN 00632036141)
2% Immunisation Against Infectious Disease	Salisbury & Begg	DoH (ISBN 011321815X)
1% Essential Statistics for Medical Practice	Rees	Chapman Hall (ISBN 0412599309)
1% The Data Sheet Compendium		British Pharmaceutical Society
1% Medical Aspects of Fitness to Drive	Gardner	Medical commission on driving and accident prevention
1% Sports Injuries 1–3	Peters & Ronstrom	Geigy Press

Table 11.1: Continued

Subject area/title	Author	Identification
Other clinical areas		
1% Geriatric problems in GP	Wilcock *et al.*	Oxford University Press (ISBN 0192613138)

Notes: this list contains many of the GP 'essentials' (BNF, Data Sheet Compendium, Medical Aspects of Fitness to Drive, Immunisation book, etc.). It also contains a few specialist books in areas that need to be covered in the practice library.

Subject area/title	Author	Identification
General recommended reading		
2% Families and How to Survive Them	Cleese & Skinner	Cedar Press
1% Life and How to Survive It	Cleese & Skinner	Cedar Press
1% I Never Promised You a Rose Garden	Green	Holt, Rhinehart & Winston
1% On Death and Dying	Kübler-Ross	Touchstone (ISBN 0684839385)
1% On Dying	Hinton	No other details found
1% A Fortunate Man	Berger & Mohr	Penguin
1% The Man who Mistook His Wife for a Hat	Sacks	Picador (ISBN 0330294911)
1% The Death of Ivan Ilyich	Tolstoy	Baltimore Penguin Books
1% The Tao of Pooh	Milne	Penguin
1% Two Short Accounts of Psychoanalysis	Freud	Pelican Books

Notes: it is immensely sad how our perception of the need to keep up to date reduces the amount of 'recreational' reading we do. This list overlaps these areas and is a challenge to trainers and registrars to broaden their minds.

A number of points emerge from this list. First, it has a long tail – only 14 books were mentioned by more than 5% of the trainers in a total of over 130 books. Second, some segments of general practice are only scantily mentioned. Screening, preventive medicine and research areas are examples. The list provides a broad indication of the books trainers find useful and is a challenge to their practice libraries.

Information technology (IT)

Most trainers are making limited use of IT facilities. It is likely that the following competencies will be required by most registrars in the near future:

1 to use IT facilities in the consultation (prescribing, note keeping, reviews, etc.)
2 to be able to access medical literature on-line (Medline, etc.)
3 to be able to send and receive e-mail communications
4 to be able to use search engines to find data on the internet
5 to use IT facilities in decision support in the consultation.

The final area above is likely to involve clinical support systems available to advise on clinical care guidelines, prescribing and referral criteria and even diagnostic decision support. Many current systems already have underused decision support systems (Emis and Mentor, the Prodigy project) which have educational potential.

Some experts believe all this will be available on mobile phone-type size, voice-activated devices within 10 years. Professor Kidd has coined the five 'golden rules' of IT:

► Rule 1: IT is *not* always the answer.
► Rule 2: IT solutions are expensive.
► Rule 3: Remember to look outside your own hard disk for a source of help.
► Rule 4: The internet is full of disorganised data *not* information.
► Rule 5: Sometimes IT is essential.

We should be aiming to learn *about* IT, learn *through* IT and learn *with* IT.

The following list is a short collection of interesting sites for the curious and committed alike. The information available is either evident within the site description or indicated below.

- American Association of Family Practitioners: http://www.aafp.org
- Arthritis: http://www.arthritisconnection.com/
- Bandolier on line (EBM information): http://www.jr2.ox.ac.uk/bandolier
- BMJ: http://www.tecc.uk/bmj/
- Canadian library of family medicine sites of interest: http://www.uwo.ca/fammed/clfn/sites.html
- Centre for Dissemination of Reviews (York): http://nhscrd.york.ac.uk
- Centre for EBM (Oxford): http://cebm.jr2.ox.uk
- CME: http://www.cme.com/
- Cochrane database (EBM information): http://www.himi.mcmaster.ca/cochrane/default.htm
- Communicable disease site: http://www.cdc.gov/
- Concensus site (guideline site): http://www.nih.gov
- Dermatology: http://derma.med.uni-erlangen.de/index_e.htm
- Doctors guide to the internet: http://www.pslgroup.com/docguide.htm
- DoH site: http://www.open.gov.uk/doh/dhhome.htm
- Family Medicine Resources: http://griffin.vcu.edu/~dimlist/
- HIV: http://hivinsite.ucsf.edu/
- Hotmail (free e-mail address): http://www.hotmail.com
- Interactive patient site: http://medicus.marshall.edu/medicus.htm
- JAMA: http://www.ama-assn.org/register/welcome.htm
- *Journal of Family Practice*: http://www.jfp.msu.edu/
- *Lancet*: http://www.thelancet.com/
- Med-E-serve (interactive CME): http://www.medeserve.com.au/
- *Medical Journal of Australia*: http://www.mja.com.au
- Medical Matrix (international resource of evaluated medical sites: http://www.medmatrix.org/index.asp
- Medline (search facility): free access as member of the BMA: type Medline in search facility

- Medline (free access): http://www.ncbi.nim.nih.gov/PubMed/
- Mental health (clinical and teaching material): http://mindset.com/cbt.html; http://mindset.com/synopsis.html
- National library of medicine: http://www.nlm.nih.gov
- North American EBM site: http://www.ohsu.edu.bicc-informatics/ebm/
- Oncolink cancer services site: http://cancer.med.upens.edu/
- Oxford University Press site: http://www.oup.co.uk/scimed
- Prevention site: http://www.ahcrp.gov/ppip/
- Pubmed (free Medline access): http://www4.ncbi.nim.nih.gov/PubMed/ebm_topics.htm
- RACGP: http://racgp.org.au
- Radcliffe Online: www.primarycareonline.co.uk
- RCGP: http://rcgp.org.edu/
- Reference site (for finding references): http://www.time.net/users/jtward/index.html
- Sports medicine – for runners: http://www.runnersworld.com – for doctors: http://www.physsportsmed.com
- Teaching – society of family medicine teachers – epulse: http://stfm.org – a GP education site that requires registration but has a lot of educational material on it.
- Travel health: http://www.cdc.gov/travel/travel.html
- 'Uncover' journal search site (journal site): http://www.carl.org/uncover
- Virtual medical centre (teaching tools): http://www-sci.lib.uci.edu/~martindale/medical.html
- Visible human project (anatomy, investigation site): http://www.nim.nih.gov/research/visible/visiblehuman.html
- Waterstones book shop on line: http://www.waterstones.co.uk
- *Which?* magazine on line: http://www.which.net
- WHO: http://www.who.ch/
- WONCA: http://www.wonca.org

The practice library

What books should a training practice have in the their library? Many trainers have asked themselves this question – usually just before a training practice accreditation visit! It is really the wrong question – what is the library for?

► to act as a reference source for the PHCT that is up to date, accessible and user friendly
► to act as a stimulus to the development of the practice and individuals
► to satisfy any external assessors.

It therefore needs to be a visible, current, evolving, stimulating and comprehensive tool for the whole PHCT to use.

One method of assessing the library is shown in the Appendix to Chapter 10. This is a tool used by visiting teams on training accreditation visits and can be used by trainers to assess their own libraries.

Trainers should consider a written library policy to cover the following areas:

► named member of PHCT in charge
► named clerical support staff
► a catalogue system that lists books by title/author/subject/date of publication (plus ISBN number/publisher, if desired)
► a defined and easily recognised filing system
► a policy for lending books and recording their whereabouts/spotting unreturned books
► a policy for periodic review of contents, i.e. for weeding out and adding to the library
► a policy on acquiring and cataloguing new books
► a budgetary policy for the library
► an advertising process to raise awareness of new material to the readership
► a process to review and audit the library policy

▶ a policy for dealing with journals (i.e. which ones/how long to be kept, etc.)

▶ a system for storing and displaying material that is difficult to classify (i.e. NHS documents, folders, videos, IT resources, tapes, etc.).

Summary comments

The wonderful thing about libraries is that they are all different. This section has confirmed that training practice libraries reflect this point. At the end of the day the value of a library is not 'bums on seats' or 'eyes on print', but quality of contents. This section has tried to facilitate the pursuit of this quality.

Appendix to Chapter 11

General reading advice

This is a copy of advice to a new registrars. It is an example of one practice's approach, provided to stimulate thought. Many of the books are described in the 'Books' section of this chapter.

GPVT reading list

There is too much to read and yet the success of your year in the practice will depend on a regular reading habit – 'So how do I start?' – read on!

This sheet should help you to develop your own reading pattern that you should continue developing throughout your career.

The list is your trainer's personal view – if you find any better books please tell them!

There are three main ways of dealing with material that you *might* read:

1 Throw it away unopened.
2 Scan the contents and *only* keep it if it contains an article you *will* read.
3 Read the entire publication.

Beware of three common traps:

1 Keeping articles you think you *should,* but probably won't read.
2 Keeping articles you are interested in and probably *don't need* to read.
3 Trying to read everything.

Using these ideas assess the material you are looking at.

Many articles contain either summaries or 'key point' sections that can be read as a guide – in many cases these cover most of the necessary information.

All of the material mentioned is available in the practice (except the *Lancet*, etc.).

1 JOURNALS

▶ *BMJ*:   most GPs either scan or read the relevant sections regularly
▶ *BJGP*:   worth scanning, particularly if doing MRCGP
▶ *Lancet*: only read by a minority
▶ *Pulse*: ⎫
▶ *GP*: ⎬ each of these three has its devotees, probably worth
▶ *Doctor*: ⎭ reading one regularly

- *Evidence Based Medicine*: early promise not really fulfilled from primary care viewpoint
- *Drugs and Therapeutics Bulletin*: read and valued by many GPs. Succinct and authoritative
- *Training Update*: ⎫
- *Practitioner*: ⎭ both of these contain useful clinical reviews and up-to-date information on training, and should be scanned for content.

There are others, but few of them are regularly read.

Other infrequent but regular publications:

- Effective health care series: detailed but useful on particular subjects
- MeReC: vary but can be helpful.

2 REFERENCE BOOKS

You need access to all these but do not really need to read them from cover to cover – at least not unless preparing for the MRCGP. They are reference books in the true sense of the phrase – you will find them useful to refer to. The following is a list of the ones available in our library – you may find others more useful. If you do, please tell us about them.

- *Immunisation Against Infectious Disease* (DASS)
- *Medical Aspects of Fitness to Drive* (Commission on accident prevention)
- A book on contraception by Guillebaud
- *MIMS*
- *British National Formulary*
- Access to a dermatology atlas
- A book on ophthalmology: *What Shall I Do?* (Kaski and Daly); *The Unquiet Eye* (Bron); *The Eye in General Practice* (Jackson and Finley)

- A book on practical general practice (Khot and Polmear)
- A book on interpretation of tests: *Pathinterp* (Warwick, IMS Publishers); *Pathognosis* (Warwick, IMS Publishers); RCR guidelines
- A 'general medical' text for reference: *Merck Manual*; McWhinney
- A copy of the *Pulse* 'Blue Book'
- Terms of service (Health authority)
- The 'Red Book' (Health authority)
- The local regional guides (summative assessment, general advice, etc.).

3 SUBJECT BOOKS

These are intended for reference/study – for the MRCGP purposes there are other books besides this list of which you should be *aware* – don't treat it as a definitive glossary!

- *Geriatric Problems in Practice* (part of the Oxford series)
- *Management in Practice* (part of the Oxford series)
- *Locomotor Disability in Practice* (part of the Oxford series)
- *Women's Problems in Practice* (part of the Oxford series)
- *Modern Obstetrics in GP* (part of the Oxford series)
- *Oxford Registrar Pocket GP Guide* (part of the Oxford series)
- A book on the NHS: *General Practice: Essential Facts* (Jones and Menzies, published by Radcliffe Medical Press)
- A book on alternative therapies: *Complementary Medicine: an integrated approach* (Lewith)
- A book on care of the dying: *Living with Dying* (Saunders); *Domiciliary Terminal Care* (Doyle)
- A book on modern management of skin conditions
- A book on screening: *The Screening Handbook* (Fry)
- A minor surgery book including soft tissue injections

- A book on child health: *Child Health Surveillance Handbook* (2e) (Hall)
- A book on guidelines
- A book on psychiatry in primary care: *A Guide to Psychiatry in Primary Care* (Casey)
- A book on running the practice: *Making Sense of General Practice* (Ellis); *Running a practice* (Bolden *et al.*)
- *ABC of ENT* (BMA Books)
- *ABC of 1–7* (BMA Books)
- *Medical Evidence for SSP/SMP and Social Security Incapacity Benefit Purposes* (DSS)
- Books to prompt education: GP series pocket guides; CASE series (Dundee University GP Education Department)
- RCGP publications – occasional papers/policies/reports
- Books on communication: *The Doctor's Communication Handbook* (2e) (Tate); *The Inner Consultation* (Neighbour); *The Doctor–Patient Relationship* (Brown and Freeling)
- A book on audit
- An MRCGP book.

WHERE DO I START?

Identify *regular* times when you *will* read – even if it is only for 10 minutes or so. Make it enjoyable, i.e. create variety – short, sharp articles in small time slots, longer 'in-depth' reading when you are more relaxed and have time.

When you look at a journal, use the following guide to scan the contents:

- Quickly look at the contents – anything interesting? Why is it interesting?
- Look at the interesting section? Read the summary, read the conclusion or key points boxes? Is it still going to help you to read it? Still interested?

- ▶ Look at the methodology and generalisability to your situation? Still good?
- ▶ Will it change what you do?
- ▶ If you've got this far you've probably read it!

Now books:

- ▶ Start with a general book – *The Doctor–Patient Relationship* or *The Doctor's Communication Handbook* (2e).
- ▶ Look for a clinical management book – *Practical GP*.
- ▶ Find the reference books.
- ▶ Start to identify areas you need to improve.

Ask for help!

Practice library assessment form

CONTENT

The content is the most important aspect of a practice library. The relevance and publication date of material is more important than quantity. Does the library have the following? (categories can be amended to suit the requirements of individual schemes).

	Yes	*No*	*Date of publication*
Medical textbooks			
Medicine			
Paediatrics			
Surgery			
Obstetrics			
Minor surgery			
Skin			
Ophthalmology			
ENT			

	Yes	*No*	*Date of publication*
Orthopaedics/ rheumatology			
Therapeutics			
Psychiatry			
Gynaecology			
Contraception			
Geriatrics			
General practice texts			
Administration/ management			
The consultation			
Overview text			
Prevention/screening			
Training/teaching material			
MRCGP text			
Terminal illness			
Chronic illness			
Ethics/philosophy text			

Journals
BMJ
BJGP
Update
Lancet
DTB
EBM
Other

Are they up to date and filed in order?	Yes/No
Are indexes available?	Yes/No
Any audiovisual material available?	Yes/No
Are there any other relevant pamphlets/ reprints?	Yes/No

Will the material help registrars develop
critical reading skills?   Yes/No

What is the most recent book
acquired? ....

Why was it bought? ....

Does the library meet the regional
recommendations?   Yes/No

CONTENT ASSESSMENT

Poor				Adequate					Good
1	2	3	4	5	6	7	8	9	10

ORGANISATION

This is of secondary importance although good organisation will facilitate more efficient use of the library content.

Is the collection accessible in one unit?   Yes/No
Is there a system for identifying borrowed/
outlying books?   Yes/No
Is there an index of material held?   Yes/No
Does this index have author/date published/
title details listed?   Yes/No
Is there a named librarian?   Yes/No
Is there any indication of budgeting?   Yes/No

How is this budget used? ....

Who is the named librarian? ....
(ideally the trainer should have a pivotal role in the
organisation)

Does the library have an internet connection? Yes/No
Does the library have Medline access? Yes/No
Are there any other useful IT resources
available? Yes/No

Does the trainer have knowledge of other
local or national library resources? Yes/No

ORGANISATIONAL ASSESSMENT

Poor				Adequate					Good
1	2	3	4	5	6	7	8	9	10

CHAPTER 12

Troubleshooting: how do trainers deal with the 'difficult' registrar?

Difficult: not easy; hard to perform; obscure; involved; hard to get on with; troublesome; stubborn

Penguin English Dictionary

Introduction

Most trainers are motivated to train by a desire to contribute to professional development, for the challenge and the stimulation and for the personal gains in terms of satisfaction, confidence and CME. A difficult registrar can undermine these motivations rapidly. What advise is on offer to help in this situation? The most common pieces of advice from trainers had three main themes: first, aim to identify problems as early as possible; second, share the problem with your partners, your fellow trainers, the regional advisors *and* the registrar as early as possible; and third, document *everything*. Some regional offices produce advice booklets and these should be read in conjunction with the following thoughts.

The problems

Prevention is better than cure, or so they say. What patterns of difficult registrar can we identify?

- the overconfident registrar
- the registrar who is always right (unable to compromise)
- the registrar trained overseas
- the registrar with poor English language skills
- the registrar with rigid, fixed belief systems (usually religious)
- the abrasive registrar (usually with staff)
- the very shy registrar
- the clinically incompetent registrar
- the registrar with exceptionally poor communication skills
- the 'reluctant' registrar, i.e. simply doing time with no drive or enthusiasm
- the 'distracted' registrar, i.e. one with severe outside pressures
- the 'unhappy' registrar, i.e. away from home, family, etc.
- the 'unaware' registrar, i.e. no personal insight
- the registrar with a drug problem
- the excellent registrar who challenges and extends the trainer
- the indecisive registrar
- the impaired registrar (mental or severe physical impairment)
- the 'business' registrar, i.e. has other business-type commitments
- the 'odd' or 'angry' registrar.

Approaches

Trainers should ask themselves the following questions:

- Why does there appear to be a problem?

- What objective evidence do I have to support this?
- Why is the registrar behaving this way?
- Why am I reacting this way?
- How can I best handle myself?
- How can I best handle this person in this situation?

The trainer needs to recognise the need for action that should aim to produce insight and a long-term outcome. The trainer has to recognise that change is solely within the power of the registrar. Trainers should consider the following steps:

1 Assume a win–win solution is possible (*see* Chapter 1).
2 Plan to sit down together in a relaxed environment with plenty of time.
3 Consider planning this discussion within the context of a regular review.
4 Identify the problem with an objective approach and evidence to back up observations. Keep observations about behaviour separate from the person.
5 Listen uncritically to the registrars concerns/ explanation and observations.
6 Try and clarify a mutual understanding of the reasons for the situation.
7 Don't aim to criticise or punish. Accept apologies.
8 Explore the registrar's options only suggesting your own if necessary.
9 Make it easy to agree.
10 Check the emotional state of the registrar and act if necessary.
11 Check your own emotional state and act if necessary.

There are three possible styles for dealing with the difficult person. None is ideal and each is useful in the correct context.

- *The nurturing parent or friendly helper*: very supportive, helpful and accepting. Potentially too gentle, avoiding flaw recognition, giving dishonest feedback and lowering standards.

- *The structuring parent or tough boss*: firm, setting good rules and definite limits. Tends to be strict, critical and sarcastic leaving the registrar defensive and depressed.
- *The logical thinker*: uses a practical and realistic problem solving approach. Tends to be cold and unaware of feelings.

It can be useful for trainers to consider their natural style and whether variations of this style may be helpful to different registrars. If the interaction has been successful, trainers often comment on a rapid resolution of the problem and an improvement in their relationship with the registrar. The latter often involves more self-disclosure and more self-awareness. However, the process can be quite anxiety provoking for all parties.

Any trainer who is having problems with a registrar should discuss this with fellow trainers and the local course organiser, and should consider involving the regional advisor. It is imperative to keep comprehensive records in this situation. These should document the evidence for concern and all actions taken to deal with the problem.

Summary comments

The difficult registrar can present a real challenge to the training practice. Achieving a change in these situations is not easy but can be one of the high points of training. In many cases it will be a long and emotionally taxing experience. Some planning and forethought may reduce the burden.

CHAPTER 13

Tips and tricks (trainers' uncut educational gems): what other ideas did trainers have to share?

… ideas are born from life

Weizsacker

Introduction

When completing the questionnaire, many trainers added comments and shared thoughts that do not fit easily into the other sections. It would be a shame to lose them, so here they are; some are the after dinner mints of the manual (short and sweet), others are the cheese and port (food for thought and appreciation) and some perhaps even the party games (frivolous and fun).

Trainers' educational gems

ABCD

This is an aide-mémoire to think about when facing an ill child. It helps to analyse the components of the seriously ill child presentation:

▶ **A**lertness, **A**tony, **A**ge-related responsiveness
▶ **B**reathing (especially recession)
▶ **C**irculation, **C**rying (whimper), **C**oncern (parental)
▶ **D**iet (i.e. reduced or none), **D**ehydration.

It can form the basis for a tutorial or analysis of a clinical situation (modified from Hewson and Gollan 1995).

Admission

Many registrars have negative feelings about admitting patients that have their roots in the derogatory comments made by hospital doctors on the receiving end of an admission. Discussing this issue can help, but the following four-point 'reasons for admission' can be a useful means of considering the issues:

▶ Medical: the patient's medical condition alone justifies admission.
▶ Social: the social situation at home, combined with the clinical problem, makes admission advisable.
▶ Organisational: although this situation could be managed at home the system cannot meet the needs of this patient (e.g. your home physiotherapy service is unavailable in this area).
▶ Personal: your personal feelings or circumstances make managing this patient at home difficult (e.g. you are going on holiday tonight).

Assumptions

This a useful way of challenging a registrar who makes assumptions inappropriately. Write down the word assume and then divide it as shown: ASS / U / ME, i.e. assume makes an ASS out of U and ME!

BATHE and ICE

This is a simple reminder of how to inquire about possible psychological elements of a problem. It is useful for the 'medical model' registrar.

- ▸ Ask about **B**ackground. What is happening in your life currently?
- ▸ Ask about **A**ffect. How do you feel?
- ▸ Ask about **T**roubles. Is anything worrying you at the moment?
- ▸ Ask about **H**andling. How are you managing at the moment?
- ▸ Show **E**mpathy. That sounds hard. It must be difficult.

The ice simply adds **I**deas (Why do you think this has happened?), **C**oncerns (Have you any other questions?) and **E**xpectations (What can we do about this?).

CAGE

This is a screening tool to help registrars enquire about alcohol consumption. Has anyone **C**riticised the patient about their consumption; does it **A**nnoy them when people enquire about their consumption; do they feel **G**uilty about their intake; and do they drink early in the morning (**E**ye-opener)? Two or more positive answers suggest alcohol dependence.

Chunk, Chop, Check

This is a brief reminder of how to share information. Put the information into related chunks or blocks, chop these into bite-sized short sentences, and check where they have gone – ask the patient!

Disney theory

Walt Disney apparently had three rooms which he used to develop his cartoons. The 'Dream' room where any ideas were allowed with no restraint (i.e. everything is possible). The 'Solution' room where answers to each problem were considered assuming limitless resources (i.e. all problems have solutions). Finally the 'Reality' room where a product must emerge. These states can be used to consider problems and help by encouraging breadth of thought and dropping the baggage of past restraints.

Heartsink patients

The five categories of heartsink patients can form the basis of an interesting tutorial – particularly with the added concept that it may be heartsink doctors who get heartsink patients.

- Manipulative help rejecter
- Entitled demander
- Dependent clinger
- Self-destructive denier
- Persistent non-responder.

Health economics

The concepts of QALYs (quality-adjusted life years) and HYEs (health-year equivalents) can form the basis of a tutorial.

Juggling

At some stage in the year the registrar has to face choices. Making choices often involves dropping options. An interesting way of exploring this is to use a set of juggling balls with labels for the choices. As a particular choice is literally dropped the registrar's feelings can be explored. Even good jugglers can be made to drop the balls!

Kipling's six wise men

> I keep six honest serving men
> (They taught me all I knew);
> Their names are What and Why and When
> And How and Where and Who

This can be used to encourage a more analytical approach in the 'poetic'!

Management tools

Surveys have indicated that most registrars have only limited understanding of practice management at the end of the year.
Consider:

▶ going through last year's accounts with them (practice and personal)
▶ running a mock job application process at the end of the year selecting a practice from the *BMJ*, writing a mock letter of application, a reply and a mock interview (even a mock rejection!)
▶ showing and discussing the practice agreement with the registrar
▶ trying to give him or her a real area of responsibility, i.e. ordering some equipment, looking at the DDA system, etc.

Minor surgery tips

1 You can practise excision of cysts by pushing an olive under loosened pork skin (get a knuckle from the

butcher) and trying to excise it without marking the olive (i.e. you wouldn't have broken the cyst).

2 Make a video of your own/your partner's minor operations to use in demonstration of technique.

3 Xanthelasma can be treated with 20% or 40% potassium hydroxide. The lower strength is painted on very carefully (to avoid the eye) with a cotton wool bud. The lesion turns a dramatic white and then involutes. The treatment can be repeated with the higher strength if necessary.

4 Produce a list of procedures to be 'ticked' off as they are covered, i.e.:

Procedure	Registrar confident doing this observed	Registrar confident doing this alone
IGTN wedge	Observed Sep 98	Oct 98
Sebaceous cyst excision	Previous experience Observed Sep 98	Sep 98

This tends to ensure most procedures are kept in mind and covered.

5 The RCGP website contains details of a minor surgery CD-ROM that illustrates all the common techniques.

NESCAFE

This is a mnemonic to encourage critical prescribing:

- Is the drug   **N**ecessary?
- Is the drug   **E**ffective?
- Is the drug   **S**afe?
- Is the drug   **C**ost-effective?
- Are there any   **A**lternatives?
- What   **F**ollow-up is indicated?
- Does the drug have any   **E**xtra features?

Patient problem pie

This is a system for analysing the possible learning requirements generated by a patient presentation. The registrar
is encouraged to produce a breakdown of the skills and
knowledge required to tackle the problem using three
areas: cognitive, affective and psychomotor. The constituent elements of each of these areas are analysed and
learning needs derived from this. The 'pie' is illustrated
in Figure 13.1.

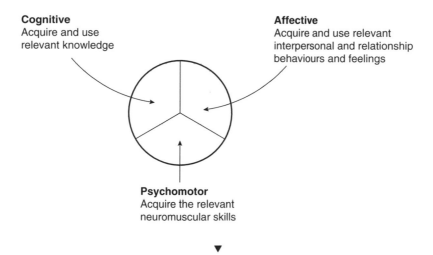

Cognitive
Acquire and use
relevant knowledge

Affective
Acquire and use relevant
interpersonal and relationship
behaviours and feelings

Psychomotor
Acquire the relevant
neuromuscular skills

Figure 13.1: Patient problem pie.

PLISSIT

This is a counselling aide-mémoire to act as a guide for
the GP 'amateur' counsellor:

▸ **P**   **P**ermission from the patient for the doctor to
adopt this role is often implied but really should
be considered carefully by the doctor.

▸ **LI**   the giving of **L**imited amounts of **I**nformation is appropriate.

▸ **SS**   the doctor should carefully consider any **S**pecific **S**uggestions that they may offer, i.e. are they appropriate?

▸ **IT**   the GP should consider if this patient needs **I**ntensive **T**reatment, e.g. referral should be considered.

Prevention: the 'Stages of Change Model' (Prochaska and DiClemente 1986)

This is a five-stage model to help link prevention activity to the patient's motivational stage.

▸ Stage 1: Pre-contemplation: raise awareness by feeding back the patient's views aiming to produce cognitive dissonance (i.e. make them uncomfortably aware).

▸ Stage 2: Contemplative: reflect positive statements and encourage solutions for change.

▸ Stage 3: Action: provide information, choices, goal setting, active support.

▸ Stage 4: Maintenance: provide follow-up (personal, group, community, etc.). Reinforce behaviours, outcomes and strategies to prevent relapse.

▸ Stage 5: Relapse: analyse reasons for relapse; support and encourage.

Prevention: the '4A' model

This is a simple aide-mémoire to encourage screening activity in the consultation. Remember to **A**sk, **A**dvise, **A**ssist and **A**rrange follow-up (from the RACGP).

Prevention: the Canadian assessment scheme

This is a simple lettering scheme that grades the evidence-based reliability of the area looked at:

A Good evidence available to support this action.
B Fair evidence to support this action.
C Equivocal or incomplete evidence to support this action.
D Some evidence to suggest this action is not advisable.
E Good evidence to suggest this action is not indicated.

An increasing number of publications are beginning to use this system to aid clinicians. It has been applied to screening procedures and drug use particularly.

Prevention

Try this on your 'classical' registrar. Aesculapis had two daughters: Panacea (the goddess of cure) and Hygiena (the goddess of prevention). How do you think they related to each other and why? (They continually fought!) This can provide a stimulus for discussion about the tensions between curative and preventative medicine – nothing is new!

Props and stunts

Change the tutorial environment: go for a walk! Show some pictures: Michelangelo's *Pieta* to illustrate releasing the inner learner; Escher's work to discuss perspectives; Dali's work to talk about time, space and stress; Constable to illustrate tranquillity, etc. Use some poetry or quotations, etc.

Settling a registrar in

The following touches were suggested by one trainer:

- Make sure a nameplate is up on his or her room (give it to him or her when he or she leaves).
- Ask them to bring in some pictures in the first week.
- Give them a box of equipment and the important paperwork and the time to go and put it in their room where they want it.
- Put a brief description on the notice board telling patients a bit about them.

'Sieving'

This is a technique designed to increase awareness of the implications of primary care behaviours. It expands the horizons of the registrar and is useful MRCGP preparation. The implications of a particular action are put through a series of 'sieves' to see if there are any potential effects. The sieves may vary from problem to problem. An example is shown in Table 13.1.

Table 13.1: 'Sieves'

Patient's sieve	Doctor's sieve	Practice sieve	Management sieve	Other sieves
Patient	Doctor	Finance	Finance	Finance
Primary carers	Partners	Staff	Trusts	Drug companies
Families	Colleagues	PHCT	Secondary care	
Communities	Profession	Primary care groups	Health authority Government	

SOAP

This established system is useful for the registrar who has problems note keeping or structuring his or her thoughts:

- ► **S**ubjective: what did the patient say?
- ► **O**bjective: what evidence of ill health have I elicited?
- ► **A**ssessment: what do we make of the situation?
- ► **P**lan: what are we going to do?

Stress at work

1 The three 'Cs': if present these reduce levels of stress: **C**ontrol, **C**ommitment, **C**hallenge.
2 The three 'horizons': have three horizons to look at, each with the promise of a positive experience, i.e. make plans that you look forward to in the short-, intermediate- and long-term future.
3 The three 'times' table: stress can be reduced by having:
   - time for oneself
   - time for a friend/mate
   - time for a group (not usually medical).
4 Enjoy the now: recognise that the only real time is now – the past is gone and the future is unpredictable. Look for satisfaction in every situation and now.
5 Know yourself: if you can achieve this you can manage your own resources to better effect:
   Know your moods
   Know your personality
   Know your transferences (i.e. feelings that dredge up hidden meanings)
   Know your 'gotchas' (i.e. actions/situations/words that get to you)
   Know your agendas (i.e. what you want)
   Know your current stress level
   Know your actual communication skill level
   Know your visionary dust depth (How long is it since you dusted your dreams?)
   Know when to get help.
6 The '10 commandments' of stress reduction, i.e.
   Thou shalt not be perfect or even try to be.
   Thou shalt not try to be all things to all people.

Thou shalt leave things undone which ought to have been done.
Thou shalt not spread thyself too thin.
Thou shalt learn to say NO.
Thou shalt not feel guilty.
Thou shalt schedule time for thyself and thy friends.
Thou shalt switch off and do nothing regularly.
Thou shalt be boring, untidy, inelegant and unattractive at times.
Thou shalt be thine own best friend and never thine own worst enemy.

Threshold of diagnosis recognition graph

This is a concise way of illustrating the problems of diagnosis in GP, i.e. different diseases look the same early on, need different levels of safety netting depending on their pattern of progression and the threshold of presentation, and recognition varies from person to person and doctor to doctor, i.e. life's a bitch!

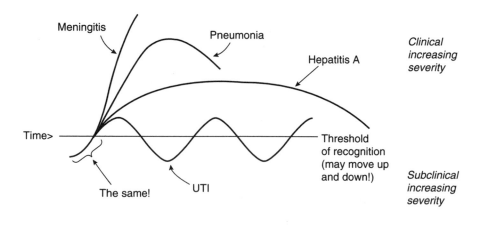

Figure 13.2: Threshold of diagnosis recognition.

'Tiering'

This is a technique used to increase a registrar's awareness of the rationale behind their behaviour in practice. It is also useful in preparation for the MRCGP. For a particular action the learner runs through the following tiered hierarchy, going as far down the tiers as they think necessary or possible:

- Tier 1: What is your normal practice?
- Tier 2: What is your peer group normal practice?
- Tier 3: What are the current professional views in this area?
- Tier 4: Is there a relevant consensus document or set of guidelines?
- Tier 5: Is there published evidence of relevance?
- Tier 6: Can you name the evidence?
- Tier 7: Can you comment on the quality of the evidence?
- Tier 8: Can you provide detail of the specific literature?

The 'virtual' surgery

All trainers are familiar with random case analysis and selective case analysis. An interesting variation is to write a brief 'virtual' surgery list covering the area of your tutorial theme, i.e. if you are looking at asthma write brief presentations for about 10 patients covering the points you feel relevant/difficult.

Summary comments

This list could probably be endless. It illustrates the breadth and depth of approach trainers use. These approaches will continue to multiply and evolve to the benefit of the registrars. We think this is best summed up by two comments trainers made on the questionnaire:

▶ 'I'm not sure if I'm a good trainer but I think I'm a good educational resource.'
▶ 'I have never got it quite right: is this the challenge or am I just crap!'

► APPENDIX A

Learner-based self-confidence rating lists

Wolverhampton Grid

This is a lengthy list, its major advantage being comprehensiveness. It also contains suggestions for topic discussion in each area. The grid was revised by Black Country trainers at their annual residential workshop in 1999. The revised grid can be downloaded from the MED-WEB Birmingham University website. All of these types of assessment grids need regular review if the aim is comprehensive cover. They do attempt to measure skills confidence as well as knowledge.

Notes on use

THE GENERAL PRACTICE YEAR

(The Wolverhampton Grid, Version 3 1999)

The answers to the enclosed questions are intended to assist you and your trainer establish a baseline of your past experience at both undergraduate and postgraduate levels, and will help you develop an educational programme. Repeating the process at intervals will help to evaluate your progress over the registrar year.

Prepared for
The Black Country Trainers Annual Workshop, Bromsgrove 1999.

SECTION A

This section outlines your experience and interests to date.

Registrar Number ....

Name ....

Address ....

....

Name of your trainer ....

Medical school ....

Year of qualification ....

Higher degrees, diplomas, etc. ....

PREVIOUS EXPERIENCE

Pre-registration   1 ....

                         ....

                         2 ....

                         ....

                         ....

Other posts with   1 ....

details of   ....

experience   2 ....

gained   ....

                         3 ....

                         ....

                         4 ....

                         ....

                         5 ....

                         ....

                         6 ....

                         ....

Special interests   ....
....
....
....

Details of   ....
projects/special   ....
experience   ....
(e.g. electives)   ....
....

SECTION B

We have attempted to compile a very complete list. You cannot expect to feel confident in all of these areas, and many may be inappropriate to your own practice.

SCORING THE INVENTORY

Tick the appropriate column for your knowledge or experience of the condition in General Practice.

> **N** = **no experience and no confidence**
> **L** = **limited experience, possibly only at undergraduate level, but little confidence**
> **S** = **some postgraduate experience, but not fully confident in general practice**
> **C** = **confident to deal with the condition in general practice**
> **Comments**

CONTENTS

CURRICULUM OVERVIEW

General practice

1	**The consultation**	Models of the consultation/Consultation skills/Telephone
	Primary healthcare team	How a team functions/Roles of primary healthcare team members/Nurse practitioners
	Health promotion	Current UK screening programmes/Mental health promotion/Motivating the change to a healthy lifestyle
2	**Prescribing**	Controlled drugs/PACT/Generic and repeat prescribing/Interactions and adverse reactions/Prescribing in special groups/Compliance/Antibiotic resistance/Addiction
	Emergencies in general practice	Resuscitation/Emergency bag/Triage/Dealing with violence
3	**Chronic disease management**	Protocols/Patient literature/Specific diseases care models/Audit
	Complementary medicine	The range available/The relationship with mainstream medicine/Registration and training
	Transcultural medicine	Cultural expectations of medicine/Body language/Death

Personal development		MRCGP examination/ The role of our College/ DRCOG and other diplomas/Balancing personal and professional life

Clinical medicine

7	**Women's health**	Gynaecological examination and procedures/ Menstruation problems/ Vaginal discharge, pain and bleeding/ Menopause/Infertility/ Gynaecological malignancies/ Preconception and maternity care/Postnatal mental health/ Miscarriage/ Family planning/ Emergency contraception/ Unwanted pregnancy/ Well women screening/ Psychosexual problems
8	**Paediatrics**	Examination and developmental assessment of children and babies/ Recognising the ill child/ Paediatric resuscitation/ Neonatal and infant problems/ Common diseases/Serious diseases of children in GP/ Conditions not to be missed/Chronic disease in children/

		Aortic aneurysm/Peripheral vascular disease/ Carotid stenosis
11	**Respiratory medicine**	Peak flow meter/ Spirometry/Oxygen therapy in the home/ Respiratory emergencies/ Respiratory infections, acute and chronic COPD/Asthma/ Sarcoidosis/Alveolitis/ Malignancy/Pulmonary embolus/Occupational lung disease
12	**The nervous system**	Examining the nervous system and assessing intellectual function/ Headache/Paraesthesia/ 'Turns'/ Epilepsy/Parkinson's disease/Strokes and TIA/ Amaurosis fugax/ Multiple sclerosis/Motor neuron disease/ Guillain Barré syndrome/ Peripheral neuropathy/ Neurological symptoms in systemic disease
13	**Gastrointestinal system**	Oral disease/Oesophageal disease/Stomach cancer/ Dyspepsia, ulceration and *Helicobacter pylori*/ Jaundice/Gall bladder disease/Hepatitis/ Pancreatitis/Pancreatic neoplasia/ Inflammatory bowel diseases/Irritable bowel/

19	**Endocrine system disease**	Diabetes: diagnosis/ management of blood sugar/complication screening/Diabetes emergencies/ Thyroid: hypo/ hyperthyroidism/Goitre/ Carcinoma/ Addison's disease/ Cushing's disease/Pituitary disease
20	**Haematology**	Anaemia/Leukaemias/ Lymphoma/Myeloma/ Sickle cell disease/Thalassaemia/ Disorders of platelets
21	**Palliative care**	Symptom control/Syringe drivers/Issues/The dying child/Psychological, cultural, religious and ethnic issues in death
22	**Infections and infestations**	Notification of infectious diseases/ Childhood infections/ Bacterial/Viral/Parasitic infestations/ Monilia/Gastroenteritis/ Leptospirosis/Lyme disease
23	**Travel medicine**	Vaccination schedules for travel/Advice for patients/ Important imported infections
24	**Minor surgery**	Getting on the minor surgery list/'Item of service' fees/ Local anaesthesia/Suturing/ Histology/ Aspirating/Injecting/

25 **Miscellaneous**

Incision/Excision/
Cryosurgery/
Health and safety and
medico-legal aspects of
minor surgery
Genetic counselling/
Myalgic encephalomyelitis/
Sports medicine/
Occupational medicine

The consultation

Assess your knowledge or experience of the following in general practice:

	N	L	S	C	Comments
Models of health and illness					
Models of the consultation: 　Neighbour 　Pendleton 　Others					
The doctor/patient relationship					
Consulting on the telephone					
Breaking bad news					
The hidden agenda					
Difficult or failing consultations					
Managing the aggressive patient					
Chaperoning					
Heartsink patients					
Time management					
The medical record					
Non-verbal communication					
Ethnic issues					
The consultation as therapy					
Motivating change					
Assessing your own consultations					

The primary healthcare team

Assess your knowledge of the following in general practice:

	N	L	S	C	Comments
The role of each professional in the primary healthcare team					
Nurse practitioners, their role and training					
How teams work together					
Delegation and work sharing					
Training and education					
The role of leader					

Health education and preventive medicine

Assess your knowledge of the following in general practice:

	N	L	S	C	Comments
Team members and roles					
Motivating patients to change to a healthier lifestyle					

Screening:
    Ethics and Wilson's criteria
    Current UK programmes					

Accident prevention					
Psychological health					

Prescribing

Assess your knowledge of the following in general practice:

	N	L	S	C	Comments
Regulations for FP10 and private scripts					
Prescribing controlled drugs The drug register					
BNF Drug tariff PACT data Prescription Pricing Authority					
Generic prescribing					
Repeat prescribing					
Over-the-counter drugs					
Giving IV or IM injections					

	N	L	S	C	Comments
Interactions between commonly used drugs					
Drug adverse reactions					
Expert computerised prescribing aids					
Prescribing in special groups: – elderly – children – pregnant or breast-feeding – renal and liver disease – patients on warfarin – addicts – suicide risks					
Addiction to prescribed medication					
Compliance					
Antibiotic resistance					

Topics for discussion (suggestions for use with trainer)

- The role of prescribing as part of the consultation
- The place of placebos
- What happens to your prescription after the patient hands it to the pharmacist?
- Role of the pharmacist
- Nurse prescribing
- The NHS response to expensive new drugs
- Dealing with pharmaceutical company representatives
- Participating in clinical trials on drugs.

Emergencies in general practice

Assess your knowledge or experience of the following in general practice:

	N	L	S	C	Comments
Resuscitation					
Emergency bag					
Coping with emergencies					
Triage					
Dealing with violence in the practice					

Chronic disease management in general practice

Assess your knowledge of the following in general practice:

	N	L	S	C	Comments
Disease specific clinics in general practice					
Protocols and structured record keeping					
Team care as a focus for planning, education and audit					
Self-help groups and voluntary agencies					
Patient literature, books, handouts					

Topics for discussion (suggestions for use with trainer)

▶ Models of care for: Diabetes
Asthma/COPD
Ischaemic heart disease
Anticoagulation
Hypertension
Rheumatoid arthritis.

Complementary medicine

Assess your knowledge of the following in general practice:

	N	L	S	C	Comments
Homeopathy					
Acupuncture					
Chiropractic and osteopathy					
Herbal and Chinese medicine					
Reflexology and aromatherapy					
The relationship with mainstream medicine					
Registration and training					

Topics for discussion (suggestions for use with trainer)
▶ When and how to refer to a complementary practitioner
▶ 'Complementary medicine should be available, open access, on the NHS.'

Transcultural medicine

Assess your knowledge of the following in general practice:

	N	L	S	C	Comments
Cultural medical differences					
Disease prevalences in ethnic communities					
Attitudes to appointments and queues					
Problems of travel					
Body language					
Death					
Effect of religion on medicine					

Medicine and the law

Assess your knowledge of the following in general practice:

	N	L	S	C	Comments
Certification: Death Cremation Fitness for work					
The coroner					
Dealing with expected and unexpected death at home					
Medical reports					
Power of attorney					
Fitness to drive					
Court attendance					
Charging fees					
Medical negligence and discipline					

Ethics

Assess your knowledge of the following in general practice:

	N	L	S	C	Comments
Living wills					
Abortion					
Euthanasia					
Confidentiality					
Consent					
The GMC and 'The duties of a doctor'					
The sick doctor					
Relationships between doctors					

Topics for discussion (suggestions for use with trainer)

► Ethical dilemmas, and how to evaluate them
► The ethics of healthcare rationing.

Social services and benefits

Assess your knowledge of the following in general practice:

	N	L	S	C	Comments
Med 3 and Med 5 regulations					
Statuary sick pay and incapacity benefits					
Benefits for the disabled					
Benefits for the unemployed					
Roles of social workers					

Audit and research

Assess your knowledge of the following in general practice:

	N	L	S	C	Comments
The audit cycle					
Types of audit (structure/process/outcome)					
How to do an audit					
Research: types of studies and trials					
Observational research					
Sources of help and support					

Evidence-based medicine and critical reading

Assess your knowledge of the following in general practice:

	N	L	S	C	Comments
Evidence-based clinical effectiveness					
Understanding the statistics used in journals					
Critical reading					

Topics for discussion (suggestions for use with trainer)

▶ Which publications should a GP read?
▶ Current initiatives to ensure effective care in general practice
▶ Why do research, and how to get started.

Information technology and the internet

Do you have experience in using the following?

	N	L	S	C	Comments
Medline					
CD-ROM-based textbooks, e.g.: – *Oxford Text Book of Medicine* – eBNF					
CD-ROM evidence base: Cochrane York					
E-mail					
The internet					

Health service organisation, structure and commissioning

Assess your knowledge of the following in general practice:

	N	L	S	C	Comments
Models of purchasing healthcare					
The health authority and NHS trusts					
National organisations (GMC, GMSC, NHSE)					
Local bodies (LMC, health authorities, CHC, MAAG)					
Primary care groups/trusts					
Cost effectiveness NICE Clinical governance					

The business of general practice

Assess your knowledge of the following in general practice:

	N	L	S	C	Comments
Terms and conditions of service The Red Book					
General practitioner remuneration					
The meaning of partnership					
Funding premises					
Personal finance, pensions and tax					
The business plan					
Interviewing					
Managing the out-of-hours commitment					
The practice manager's role					
Staff management and training Employment law					
Health and Safety at Work Act/ COSHH					
NHS complaints system					

Career and personal development

Assess your knowledge of the following in general practice:

	N	L	S	C	Comments
The MRCGP examination					
The role of our Royal College					
DRCOG					
Diplomas in specialist areas					
Masters degrees in education or medical science					

	N	L	S	C	Comments
Criteria for inclusion on minor surgery and obstetric lists					
Continuing medical education					
Professional development					
The balance of personal and professional life					

Women's health

How confident are you with the following clinical skills?

	N	L	S	C	Comments
Breast examination					
Pelvic examination/use of speculum					
Taking of cervical smears					
Removal of cervical polyps					
Insertion/removal of IUCDs					
Removal of foreign bodies from the vagina					
Fitting of contraceptive diaphragms/caps					
Insertion of hormone implants					
Endometrial biopsy					
Fitting of ring pessaries					

Assess your knowledge and ability in the following:

	N	L	S	C	Comments
Problems of menstruation					
Amenorrhoea					
Premenstrual syndrome					
Vaginal discharge					
Vaginal prolapse					
Dyspareunia					
Menopause and HRT					
Vulval disorders					
Abnormal vaginal bleeding					
Gynaecological malignancies					
Psychosexual problems					
Sexuality					
The abused woman					

	N	L	S	C	Comments
Preconception care					
Antenatal care: – criteria for booking – screening fetal abnormalities – rhesus factor					
Intrapartum care/home births					
Postnatal care					
Breast-feeding					
Postnatal mental health					

	N	L	S	C	Comments
Miscarriage					
Unwanted pregnancy and abortion					
Family planning					
Emergency contraception					
The subfertile couple					
Breast lumps and pain					
Well women screening					

Paediatrics

Assess your clinical competence with reference to:

	N	L	S	C	Comments
Examination of children and babies					
Developmental assessment					
Taking a history from a child					
Recognising the ill child: – physical – social – psychological					
Paediatric resuscitation and CPR					

Assess your ability to deal with the following conditions in general practice:

Neonatal and infant problems

	N	L	S	C	Comments
Heart murmur					
Sticky eye					
Jaundice					
Congenital defects					
The pyrexial or crying child					
Infant feeding					
Vomiting and diarrhoea					

Childhood

	N	L	S	C	Comments
Constipation					
Abdominal pain, acute and recurrent					
Failure to thrive					
Rashes					
Croup and epiglottitis					
Cough/dyspnoea/wheezing					
Headache					
Febrile convulsions					
Epilepsy					
Meningitis					
Osteomyelitis					
Paediatric orthopaedics					
Urinary tract infection					
Malignant disease in children					
Accidental poisoning					
The abused child (physical, sexual and psychological)					

Chronic health problems

	N	L	S	C	Comments
Haemophilia and the haemoglobinopathies					
Asthma					
The handicapped child and cerebral palsy					
Cystic fibrosis					
Diabetes in childhood					
Arthritis					
The family of an ill child					

Death

	N	L	S	C	Comments
Sudden infant death					
Bereavement					
Death and dying					

Psychological problems

	N	L	S	C	Comments
Enuresis/encopresis					
Behavioural development and disorders					
Bullying/school refusal					
Temper tantrums					
Learning disorders in children					
Substance abuse					
Obesity/anorexia/pica					

Adolescence

	N	L	S	C	Comments
Making care accessible to adolescents					
Puberty					
Teenage pregnancy					
Contraception					
Psychosocial issues					

Miscellaneous

	N	L	S	C	Comments
Paediatric emergencies in general practice					
Accident prevention in the home					
Immunisation					
Child care ethics and legal aspects					

Topics for discussion (suggestions for use with trainer)

► Child care legislation: The Children Act, managing suspected abuse, ethics and children
► The family in trouble
► Parenting
► Conditions easily missed in GP surgeries:
  – UTI
  – diabetes
  – abuse
  – Münchausen by proxy
  – rheumatic fever
  – cystic fibrosis
  – osteomyelitis
  – malignancies
  – heart failure
  – coeliac disease

> ► Managing minor illness in children
> ► Other child care agencies and working as a child care team.

Psychiatry

Assess your clinical competence with reference to:

	N	L	S	C	Comments
Anxiety/stress					
Obsessive–compulsive disorders					
Post-traumatic stress					
Phobia					
Grief and bereavement					
Marital problems					
Psychosexual problems					
Eating disorders: Obesity Anorexia					

	N	L	S	C	Comments
Depression					
Suicide and parasuicide: risk assessment					
Acute psychoses					
Schizophrenia					
Puerperal psychosis and depression					

	N	L	S	C	Comments

Psychiatric disease in:
  Children
  Adolescents
  Elderly					

Learning disorders					
Ethnic, cultural and social issues					

	N	L	S	C	Comments
Dementia					
Psychiatric presentations in physical disease					
Alcohol use and abuse					
Drug addiction					

	N	L	S	C	Comments
Mental Health Act					
Role of the CPN and the community mental health team					
Notification and prescribing addictive drugs					

Topics for discussion (suggestions for use with trainer)

- The acute psychiatric emergency and admission to hospital
- Caring for the family of the mentally ill patient
- The use of drugs in psychiatry and their side effects
- Counselling
- The change cycle
- Atypical presentation of psychiatric disease
- Managing and caring for the chronic mentally ill patient.

The heart and circulation

Assess your clinical competence with reference to:

	N	L	S	C	Comments
Taking a blood pressure					
Assessing the heart sounds					
The use and interpretation of the ECG					
Cardiopulmonary resuscitation					

Assess your ability to deal with the following conditions in general practice:

	N	L	S	C	Comments
Myocardial infarction					
Heart failure					
Cardiac arrhythmia					
Cardiomyopathy					
Heart valve disease					
Hypertension: Epidemiology Diagnosis Management					
Angina					
IHD prevention: Primary Secondary					
Hyperlipidaemia					
Sub-acute bacterial endocarditis					
Cardiac rehabilitation					

	N	L	S	C	Comments
Aortic aneurysm and screening					
Peripheral vascular disease					
Carotid artery stenosis					
Acute arterial occlusion					
Thromboembolism					
Varicose veins and thrombophlebitis					

	N	L	S	C	Comments
Ethnic variation and issues					
Atypical presentations of cardiovascular and cerebrovascular disease					

Topics for discussion (suggestions for use with trainer)

▶ The assessment and management of the patient presenting with:
  – chest pain
  – dyspnoea
  – syncope
  – palpitations
▶ Care of the amputee
▶ Antibiotic prophylaxis
▶ Reducing cardiovascular deaths in your community
▶ Advances in the investigation and management of IHD in secondary care.

Respiratory medicine

Assess your clinical competence with reference to:

	N	L	S	C	Comments
Peak flow meter					
Spirometry					
Use of nebulisers					

Respiratory emergencies:
   Angioneurotic oedema
   Stridor
   Status asthmaticus					

Assess your ability to deal with the following conditions in general practice:

Respiratory infections

	N	L	S	C	Comments
Tracheitis					
Acute bronchitis					
Pneumonia, including atypical					
Tuberculosis					
Opportunistic infections					

Chronic pulmonary conditions

	N	L	S	C	Comments
COPD					
Asthma					
Sarcoidosis					
Pulmonary alveolitis and fibrosis					
Bronchiectasis					

Malignancy   N L S C Comments

	N	L	S	C	Comments
Carcinoma of the bronchus					
Other malignancies of the chest					
Pulmonary secondaries					

Other conditions   N L S C Comments

	N	L	S	C	Comments
Pulmonary embolus, single and multiple					
Occupational lung disease					
Pneumothorax					
Pleural effusion					
Pulmonary manifestation of diseases of other systems					

Topics for discussion (suggestions for use with trainer)

- The investigation of a patient with:
  - wheeze
  - dyspnoea
  - cough
  - shadow on chest X-ray
  - haemoptysis
- The evidence base for the treatment of acute respiratory tract infections and the use of antibiotics
- Asthma and COPD:
  - standards of care (British Thoracic Society Guidelines)
  - organising care in general practice
- Provision of oxygen therapy in the home (oxygen concentrators).

The nervous system

Assess your clinical competence with reference to:

	N	L	S	C	Comments
Assessing intellectual function					

Examining:
   Central nervous system
   Cranial nerves
   Peripheral nerves					

Assess your ability to deal with the following conditions in general practice:

	N	L	S	C	Comments
Headache: Tension Migraine Meningitis Other infections Tumour Intra-cranial haemorrhage Temporal arteritis					
Dementia (Alzheimer's and others)					
Parkinson's disease					
Strokes and TIA/amaurosis fugax					
Epilepsy					
Differential diagnosis: fits/faints/blackouts					
Multiple sclerosis					
Motor neuron disease					
Guillain Barré syndrome					
Peripheral neuropathy					
Amnesia					
Myelopathy					
Spinal claudication					

	N	L	S	C	Comments
Muscular and neuromuscular diseases					
Neurological symptoms in disease of other systems, including cancer					

Topics for discussion (suggestions for use with trainer)

- The patient with headache
- Unravelling the problem of the patient presenting with a 'turn'
- Care of the disabled patient and their family
- Tremor.

Gastrointestinal system

Assess your ability to deal with the following conditions in general practice:

	N	L	S	C	Comments
Mouth ulcers					
Oral tumours					
Oral signs of systemic or skin disease					

	N	L	S	C	Comments
Oesophageal reflux					
Dysphagia					
Oesophageal carcinoma					

	N	L	S	C	Comments
Gastroenteritis					
Dyspepsia and peptic ulceration					
Helicobacter pylori					
Stomach cancer					
Haematemesis and melaena					

	N	L	S	C	Comments
Jaundice					
Gall bladder disease					
Hepatitis, infective and non-infective					
Pancreatitis					
Pancreatic neoplasia					

	N	L	S	C	Comments
Adult coeliac disease					
Crohn's disease					
Ulcerative colitis					
Irritable bowel syndrome					
Diverticular disease					
Ischaemic bowel					
Colon carcinoma					
Caring for the patient with a stoma					
Rectal bleeding					
Anal and peri-anal diseases					
Pruritus ani					

Topics for discussion (suggestions for use with trainer)

- Assessing the acute abdomen in general practice
- General practice management of recurrent abdominal pain
- When to request endoscopy of upper or lower gastro-intestinal tract
- Management of dyspepsia including *H. pylori*
- Screening for cancer of the colon and its early diagnosis
- Altered bowel habit
- Assessing chronic diarrhoea.

Renal and genitourinary medicine

Assess your ability to deal with the following conditions in general practice:

The kidney   N L S C Comments

	N	L	S	C	Comments
Glomerulonephritis					
Renal calculi					
Pyelonephritis					
Polycystic kidneys					
Hydronephrosis					
Renal failure and dialysis					
Renal tumours					

The bladder   N L S C Comments

	N	L	S	C	Comments
Bladder tumours					
Incontinence, male and female					
Urinary retention					
Cystitis					

The prostate   N L S C Comments

	N	L	S	C	Comments
Benign prostatic hypertrophy					
Prostate cancer					
Prostatitis					

Male genitalia

	N	L	S	C	Comments
Phimosis, balanitis and circumcision					
Painful testes					
Torsion of the testis					
Lumps in the scrotum and testes					
Impotence					
Haematospermia					

Sexually transmitted diseases

	N	L	S	C	Comments
Syphilis					
Gonorrhoea					
Non-specific urethritis					
Chlamydia					
AIDS					

Topics for discussion (suggestions for use with trainer)

- Investigating blood in the urine (macro- and microscopic)
- Investigating protein in the urine
- The use of the PSA
- Management of UTI
- Problems with catheter care.

Diseases of the ear, nose and throat

How confident are you with the following clinical skills?

	N	L	S	C	Comments
Examination of the ear, nose and throat					
ENT examination in children					
Assessing hearing (Rinne's/Weber's)					
Ear syringing					

Assess your knowledge and ability in the following:

	N	L	S	C	Comments
Deafness and hearing loss					
Tinnitus					
Vertigo					
Hearing aids and their problems					

Middle ear diseases:
   Otitis media
   Glue ear
   Otosclerosis					

Mastoiditis					
Otitis externa					
Diseases of the pinna					

Epistaxis					
Allergic and vasomotor rhinitis					
Sinus problems					
Nasal obstruction/polyps					
Injuries					
Snoring					

	N	L	S	C	Comments
The acute sore throat/quinsy					
Hoarseness and other disorders of the voice					
Dysphagia					

	N	L	S	C	Comments
Head and neck pain					
Lumps in the neck					
Head and neck malignancy					

Topics for discussion (suggestions for use with trainer)

- The dizzy patient
- The painful ear
- Assessing a patient for a hearing aid
- Role of the speech therapist
- ENT emergencies
- Advances in secondary care procedures
- Indications for tonsillectomy
- The patient with a tracheostomy.

Diseases of the skin

How confident are you with the following clinical skills?

	N	L	S	C	Comments
Describing a rash					
Taking skin scrapings					
Using a Wood's light					
Pharmacology for the skin					
Caring for people with diseases of the skin					

Assess your knowledge of, and ability to diagnose and treat the following:

	N	L	S	C	Comments
Eczema					
Psoriasis					
Acne vulgaris					
Rosacea					

	N	L	S	C	Comments
Infections: Fungal Yeasts Bacterial Viral					
Erysipelas					
Warts and verrucas					
Infestations					

	N	L	S	C	Comments
Urticaria and pruritus					
Angioneurotic oedema					
Reactions to drugs					
Occupational skin disease					

	N	L	S	C	Comments
Skin manifestations of:					
Systemic disease					
Malignancy					
Metabolic diseases					

	N	L	S	C	Comments
Diseases of the scalp and hair					
Diseases of the nails					
Benign lumps and bumps					
Skin malignancy					
Leg ulcers, causes and management					

Topics for discussion (suggestions for use with trainer)

► How to describe a rash you do not recognise
► Skin problems in childhood, adolescence and old age
► Should I prescribe a cream or an ointment, or perhaps a lotion? Vehicles in dermatology
► Uses and abuses of topical steroids in dermatology.

The eye

Assess your competence in clinical examination with reference to:

	N	L	S	C	Comments
Visual acuity and the pinhole					
Visual field					
The eyelids					
The use of the ophthalmoscope					
The eyes of children					

Assess your ability to deal with the following conditions in general practice:

	N	L	S	C	Comments
Blepharitis and infection of the eyelid					
Meibomian cysts					
Entropion and ectropion					

	N	L	S	C	Comments
Ptosis and proptosis					
Squint					

	N	L	S	C	Comments
Conjunctivitis					
Dry eye					
Foreign bodies in the eye					
Corneal abrasions, ulcers and trauma					
Herpes zoster and the eye					

	N	L	S	C	Comments
Iritis					
Glaucoma					
Lens opacities					

	N	L	S	C	Comments
Optic atrophy					
Retinal detachment					
Retinal vein thrombosis					
Retinal artery occlusion					
Senile macular degeneration					

	N	L	S	C	Comments
Retinopathy: Diabetic Hypertensive					
Medication in ophthalmology					
Eye malignancies					

Topics for discussion (suggestions for use with trainer)

▶ The eye in systemic disease
▶ The red eye
▶ Problems with contact lenses
▶ Eye problems in children
▶ The eye in the elderly
▶ Aids for the visually impaired
▶ Sudden loss of vision
▶ Flashes of light
▶ Double vision
▶ Recent advances in secondary care.

Rheumatology and orthopaedics

Assess your skills in the following:

	N	L	S	C	Comments
Differential diagnosis of joint pain					
Examining joints					
Investigating joint disorders					
Injecting and aspirating joints					

Assess your ability to deal with the following conditions in general practice:

Orthopaedics

	N	L	S	C	Comments
Low back pain					
Neck pain					
Disorders of the: Hip Knee Shoulder Foot					
Osteomyelitis					
Osteochondritis					
Bone tumours					
Sprains and strains					
Tennis elbow and other tendon disorders					
Carpal tunnel syndrome					

Rheumatology

	N	L	S	C	Comments
Rheumatoid arthritis					
Connective tissue disorders					
Tendon disorders and repetitive strain injury					
Gout					
Polymyalgia rheumatica					
Seronegative arthropathies					

Topics for discussion with trainer

▶ Investigating and diagnosing joint pain in general practice
▶ Appropriate use of imaging techniques for orthopaedic conditions

- ▶ The initial and second line pharmacological treatment of polyarthritis
- ▶ Indications for referral for orthopaedic or rheumatological opinion
- ▶ Role of physiotherapy and occupational therapy
- ▶ Role of other practitioners, such as chiropractors, osteopaths and acupuncturists.

Diseases of the endocrine system

Assess your knowledge of the following in general practice:

Diabetes	N	L	S	C	Comments
Criteria for diagnosis					
Managing the newly diagnosed patient					
Control of blood sugar Who needs insulin?					
Screening for complications					
Managing diabetic foot disease					
Microalbuminuria/Hypertension/ Lipids					
Legal/Employment/Driving implications					
Psychosocial aspects of diabetes					
Diabetes emergencies					
Causes of secondary diabetes					
Impaired glucose tolerance					

Thyroid disease

	N	L	S	C	Comments

Diagnosis, management and continuing care of:
    Hypothyroidism
    Thyrotoxicosis					

Goitre					
Carcinoma of the thyroid					

Miscellaneous

	N	L	S	C	Comments
Addison's disease/crisis					
Cushing's disease					
Reproductive endocrinology					
Pituitary disease					
Parathyroid disease					

Topics for discussion (suggestions for use with trainer)

- Investigating goitre
- Long-term care for patients with thyroid disease
- Organising care for the diabetic patient
- Infertility
- Amenorrhoea
- Abnormal puberty
- The abnormal Ca^{2+}.

Haematology

Assess your knowledge of the following in general practice:

	N	L	S	C	Comments
The anaemias					
Polycythaemia					
Leukaemias					
Lymphoma					
Myeloma					
Clotting disorders					
Sickle cell disease					
Thalassaemia					
Disorders of platelets					

Topics for discussion (suggestions for use with trainer)

- Investigation and management of anaemia in general practice
- Anaemia in pregnancy
- Early diagnosis of haemopoietic malignancies
- Purpura
- Chronic haematological disease: caring for the patient and the family
- Models of care for patients on warfarin.

Palliative care

Assess your knowledge or experience of the following in general practice:

	N	L	S	C	Comments
Palliative and terminal care					
Control of pain					
Control of other symptoms					
Using a syringe driver: drug interactions					
Teamwork in palliative care: The role of: District nurse Hospice Macmillan nurses Voluntary agencies Pain clinic Oncologist					
Psychological issues in terminal care					
The dying child					
Caring for the family					
Cultural, religious and ethnic issues in death and bereavement					

Infectious diseases and infestations

Assess your experience of the following conditions in general practice:

	N	L	S	C	Comments
Notification of infectious diseases					

Childhood infections

Childhood infections	N	L	S	C	Comments
Measles					
Mumps					
Rubella					
Chickenpox					
RSV					
Pertussis					

Bacterial infections

Bacterial infections	N	L	S	C	Comments
Staphylococcal infections					
Streptococcal infections and their sequelae					
Meningitis					
Septicaemia					
Tetanus					
Brucellosis					
Tuberculosis					

Viral infections

Viral infections	N	L	S	C	Comments
Herpes simplex					
Herpes zoster					
Influenza					
Glandular fever					
Poliomyelitis					

Parasitic infestations

Parasitic infestations	N	L	S	C	Comments
Worms					
Head lice					
Scabies					

Others

	N	L	S	C	Comments
Monilia					
Gastroenteritis					
Leptospirosis					
Lyme disease					

Travel medicine

Assess your knowledge of the following:

	N	L	S	C	Comments
Vaccination schedules for travel					
Advice for patients before and after travel					
Malaria					
Diphtheria					
Rabies					
Giardiasis					

Minor surgery

Assess your ability to deal with the following conditions in general practice:

	N	L	S	C	Comments
Minor surgery list requirements					
Required facilities					
Consent					
Role of assistant					
Procedures attracting 'item of service' fee					
Record keeping					
Histology					

Local anaesthesia					
Suturing and suture materials					

Aspirating or injecting:
   Joints
   Hydrocoeles					

Incision and drainage of abscesses					
Excision of minor lumps					
Management of ingrowing toenails					
Cryosurgery					

Discussion topics (suggestions for use with trainer)

► Health and safety aspects of minor surgery
► Medico-legal aspects of minor surgery

Miscellaneous

Assess your knowledge of the following:

	N	L	S	C	Comments
Genetic counselling					
Myalgic encephalomyelitis					
Sports medicine					
Occupational medicine					

Initial educational planning assessment form

This is designed to measure the basics that should hopefully have been covered in training prior to the GP year (but often have not) as well as opening up the agenda for the year ahead. It can be used with the registrar when devising the educational plan for the first few months.

INITIAL EDUCATIONAL PLANNING FORM

This form is designed to help us determine priorities for your teaching programme. It includes the opportunity to review your feeling about the 'basics' you have already learned as well as exploring your future learning needs.

Use the following scale to indicate your confidence levels at the end of each line and return the form to your trainer.

1 = I have little confidence in my current ability
2 = I have some confidence but the area needs more attention
3 = I am reasonably confident, with slight reservations
4 = I feel confident in this area
5 = I feel entirely confident in this area

PROCEDURES			Not confident			Very confident	
1	Swabs:	wound	1	2	3	4	5
		nasal	1	2	3	4	5
		throat	1	2	3	4	5
		vaginal	1	2	3	4	5
2	Urine:	collection	1	2	3	4	5
		dipstick tests	1	2	3	4	5
		inspection	1	2	3	4	5

		Not confident			Very confident	
3	Injection techniques:					
	IV	1	2	3	4	5
	SC	1	2	3	4	5
	IM	1	2	3	4	5
	ID	1	2	3	4	5
	sites	1	2	3	4	5
	venepuncture	1	2	3	4	5
4	Minor surgery:					
	basic dressings	1	2	3	4	5
	suturing	1	2	3	4	5
	local anaesthesia	1	2	3	4	5
5	Minor surgery (non-essential):					
	use of cryotherapy	1	2	3	4	5
	use of diathermy	1	2	3	4	5
	use of curette	1	2	3	4	5
	basic joint injections	1	2	3	4	5
	foreign body removal	1	2	3	4	5
6	Resuscitation:					
	mouth-to-mouth	1	2	3	4	5
	ECM	1	2	3	4	5
	airways/bagging	1	2	3	4	5
	basic drugs	1	2	3	4	5
	choking treatment	1	2	3	4	5
	basic first aid	1	2	3	4	5
7	Others:					
	use of peak flow meter	1	2	3	4	5
	taking an ECG	1	2	3	4	5
	audiometry	1	2	3	4	5

	Not confident			Very confident	
use of nebuliser	1	2	3	4	5
use of glucometer	1	2	3	4	5
use of vitalograph	1	2	3	4	5
catheterisation (urinary)	1	2	3	4	5

EXAMINATION SKILLS

		Not confident			Very confident	
General:	taking the temperature	1	2	3	4	5
	checking lymphadenopathy	1	2	3	4	5
	examining breasts	1	2	3	4	5
CVS:	pulses (peripheral pulses)	1	2	3	4	5
	apex beat	1	2	3	4	5
	taking BP	1	2	3	4	5
	auscultating heart	1	2	3	4	5
	checking for oedema	1	2	3	4	5
RS:	checking expansion	1	2	3	4	5
	feeling trachea	1	2	3	4	5
	percussion	1	2	3	4	5
	auscultation	1	2	3	4	5
	other tests	1	2	3	4	5
GI:	palpation	1	2	3	4	5
	feeling the liver	1	2	3	4	5
	feeling the spleen	1	2	3	4	5
	feeling the kidneys	1	2	3	4	5
	feeling the bladder	1	2	3	4	5
	percussion	1	2	3	4	5
	checking for herniae	1	2	3	4	5
	auscultation	1	2	3	4	5
	other tests	1	2	3	4	5

		Not confident			Very confident	
	doing a PR	1	2	3	4	5
	proctoscopy	1	2	3	4	5
ANC:	examining the uterus	1	2	3	4	5
	examining the fetal heart	1	2	3	4	5
Eyes:	fundoscopy	1	2	3	4	5
	everting eyelids	1	2	3	4	5
	examining the cornea	1	2	3	4	5
Ears:	otoscopy	1	2	3	4	5
Throat:	looking in the nose	1	2	3	4	5
	looking in the throat	1	2	3	4	5
	examining the neck	1	2	3	4	5
Paediatrics:						
	examining fractious children	1	2	3	4	5
	measuring height/ length	1	2	3	4	5
	measuring head circumference	1	2	3	4	5
	weighing children	1	2	3	4	5
	examining neonates	1	2	3	4	5
Genital medicine:						
	examining the scrotum/penis	1	2	3	4	5
	examining the vulva	1	2	3	4	5
	doing a VE	1	2	3	4	5

	Not confident			Very confident	
using a Simms speculum	1	2	3	4	5
using a Cuscos speculum	1	2	3	4	5
taking a smear	1	2	3	4	5
doing cervical/ HV swabs	1	2	3	4	5

Orthopaedics:
(examining joints)

hands	1	2	3	4	5
elbow	1	2	3	4	5
shoulder	1	2	3	4	5
hip	1	2	3	4	5
knee	1	2	3	4	5
feet	1	2	3	4	5

Neurology:

examining cranial nerves	1	2	3	4	5
checking reflexes	1	2	3	4	5
checking power and tone	1	2	3	4	5
checking sensation	1	2	3	4	5
cerebellar signs	1	2	3	4	5

Administration:

making clinical notes	1	2	3	4	5
writing a prescription	1	2	3	4	5
admitting patients	1	2	3	4	5
referring patients	1	2	3	4	5
use of PHCT members	1	2	3	4	5

	Not confident				Very confident
use of computers	1	2	3	4	5
use of investigations	1	2	3	4	5
use of ambulances	1	2	3	4	5

Other areas:

The opportunity to discuss and experience some activity in the following areas is also possible:

	Not confident				Very confident
complementary medicine	1	2	3	4	5
IUCDs	1	2	3	4	5
caps/diaphragms	1	2	3	4	5
GPFH (budget holding)	1	2	3	4	5
dispensing	1	2	3	4	5
staff management	1	2	3	4	5
health promotion activity	1	2	3	4	5

Notes on use:

The combined confidence rating scale (CRS)

This is a comprehensive scale developed from a number of practice-designed scales.

CHECKLIST OF SUBJECTS OF IMPORTANCE IN GENERAL PRACTICE

1 It is not claimed that this checklist is comprehensive, but it is hoped that it indicates fields in which a GP should have competence or understanding in clinical, organisational and administrative fields.

2 It is suggested that the registrar should indicate his/her degree of confidence under the various headings in the early stages of training and discuss the document with the trainer. From this, discussion subjects for tutorials, and the need for reading and other educational activities should emerge.

3 Level of confidence should be given a number on the scale from 1 to 5 where 1 equates to no confidence and 5 equates to fully confident.

4 Registrars will be required to repeat the confidence scales at designated intervals during their training and when doing this to check the entries they made on the previous forms.

5 After completion the scores of repeated CRS should be entered on a master copy.

A score is placed in the relevant column allowing the scores from subsequent assessments to be compared.

GENERAL PRACTICE

Indicate your degree of confidence on the following scale, placing a figure in the relevant column for each area.

None   Full
  0   1   2   3   4   5

	CRS1 (date)	**CRS2** (date)	**CRS3** (date)
ORGANISATION OF THE NHS HA/RHS/CHC/PCG Primary/secondary care interface Budgets			
MEDICAL BODIES LMC/GMC/BMA/GMSC			
PRIMARY HEALTHCARE TEAM Nurses Midwives Social workers CPNs Pharmacists Physiotherapists Occupational therapists Administrative staff			
THE CONSULTATION Appointment systems Consultation models Consultation mapping/tasks Difficult patients Confidentiality Complaints/risk management			

	CRS1 (date)	CRS2 (date)	CRS3 (date)
PAPERWORK			
Forms			
Records/notes			
CERTIFICATION			
Sickness certification			
Benefit claims			
Attendance allowance/DS1500			
DLA/DWA			
Death certification			
Cremation			
The coroner			
ON-CALL			
The black bag			
Cooperative arrangements			
Being on-call			
SCREENING AND PREVENTION			
Theory/principles			
Hypertension			
Cervical cytology			
Mammography			
Prostate cancer			
Bowel cancer			
TERMINAL CARE			
Symptom control			
Hospice use			
Macmillan nurses			
Bereavement/grief			
Family support			

	CRS1 (date)	CRS2 (date)	CRS3 (date)
PROFESSIONAL DEVELOPMENT			
Keeping up to date			
Research			
Audit			
Preventing burnout			
Extended professional roles			
Sick doctors			
MEDICAL TOPICS			
INFECTION			
Minor viral illnesses			
Childhood exanthemata			
PUO			
D & V			
Hepatitis A–C (and others)			
Notifiable disease			
Vaccination in adults			
Travel vaccination			
Vaccination in children			
ENT			
Catarrhal problems			
Otitis media			
Otitis externa			
Tonsillitis and tonsillectomy			
Glue ear			
Vertigo			
Ménière's syndrome			
Hay fever			
Dizziness			
Epistaxis			
Deafness			

	CRS1 (date)	CRS2 (date)	CRS3 (date)
EYES			
Examination of the eye			
Sudden visual loss			
Gradual visual loss			
The painful red eye			
Glaucoma			
Blindness/registration			
Squint			
Orthoptics			
Styes and cysts			
Cataracts			
CHEST MEDICINE			
Smoking			
COPD			
Asthma			
Lung cancer			
Fibrotic lung disease			
Sleep apnoea			
Spirometry			
Chest infections			
CVS MEDICINE			
Angina pectoris			
AMI management			
CVA/TIA			
Peripheral vascular disease			
Hypercholesterolaemia			
Heart failure			
ECG use			
OBSTETRICS			
Preconceptual care			
Antenatal care			

	CRS1 (date)	**CRS2** (date)	**CRS3** (date)
Intrapartum care			
Postnatal care			
Choice of place of delivery			
Abortion Act			
Obstetric emergencies:			
APH			
Miscarriage			
PPH			
Fetal distress			
Resuscitation of mother			
Resuscitation of newborn			
GYNAECOLOGY			
Vaginal discharge			
Infertility			
Menstrual problems			
Contraception:			
POP			
COCP			
IUCD			
Implants			
Barrier methods			
Physiological methods			
Sterilisation			
Psychosexual problems			
Incontinence			
Abnormal vaginal bleeding			
Menopause			
HRT			
Cervical smear abnormalities			
Gynaecological cancers			
Breast cancer			
Breast problems			

	CRS1 (date)	CRS2 (date)	CRS3 (date)
PAEDIATRICS			
Infant feeding			
Child health surveillance			
Developmental assessments			
Paediatric emergencies			
Febrile fits			
UTIs			
Meningitis			
Congenital birth defects			
Enuresis			
SIDS			
NAI			
Behavioural problems			
Fever management			
Childhood asthma			
CNS MEDICINE			
Epilepsy			
Migraine			
Headaches			
Parkinsonism/movement disorders			
Cerebral tumours			
Examination of the CNS system			
ORTHOPAEDICS			
OA			
RA			
LBP			
Osteoporosis			
Joint surgery			
Joint injection			
Joint examination			

	CRS1 (date)	CRS2 (date)	CRS3 (date)
PSYCHIATRY			
Mental state assessment			
Suicidal risk assessment			
Depression			
Anxiety			
Psychoses			
Mental Health Act			
Use of CMHT			
Counselling			
Simple psychotherapy			
Eating disorders			
Somatisation			
Alcohol abuse			
Drug abuse			
Acute confusion			
Dementia			
ENDOCRINOLOGY			
Diabetes mellitus			
Hyperthyroidism			
Hypothyroidism			
DERMATOLOGY			
Eczema			
Psoriasis			
Acne vulgaris			
Acne rosacea			
Leg ulcers			
Infestations			
Fungal infections			
Lumps/bumps			
Skin malignancies			
Bacterial infections in the skin			

	CRS1 (date)	**CRS2** (date)	**CRS3** (date)
Viral infections in the skin			
Diagnosis of skin disease			
GU MEDICINE			
UTIs			
Prostatic disease			
Bladder problems			
GU malignancies			
Haematuria			
Renal failure			
MINOR SURGERY			
Approval and organisation			
Suturing			
Excisions			
Cautery			
Cryocautery			
Curettage			
Injections/aspirations			
IGTNs			
THERAPEUTICS			
Controlled drug regulations			
Writing a script			
Charges/exemptions			
Budgets/PACT			
Dispensing			
Drug companies			
Formularies			
Drug interactions			
Repeat prescribing			
Computer prescribing			
Sources of information			
Assessing quality of prescribing			

	CRS1 (date)	CRS2 (date)	CRS3 (date)

COMPLEMENTARY MEDICINE
Homeopathy
Acupuncture
Osteopathy
Chiropractic medicine
Reflexology
Herbal medicines
Others

MANAGEMENT AND ADMINISTRATION

STAFF
Practice manager
Hiring and firing
Contracts/job descriptions
Budgets
Motivation

PREMISES
Owning/renting
Cost/notional rents
Financing premises
Premise management

MONEY
Income/expenditure
Private income
The Red Book (SFA)
Accounting
Tax
Partnership financial agreements

	CRS1 (date)	CRS2 (date)	CRS3 (date)
PARTNERSHIPS			
Practice agreements			
Finding a practice			
Principles of team working			
Practice meetings			
Terms of service			
Stress prevention			
Locum work			
COMPUTERS			
Day-to-day use			
Financing			
Updating			
Potential/future use			
ASSESSMENT			
VIDEO			
Consent			
Practical use			
SUMMATIVE ASSESSMENT			
Principles			
Audit/alternatives			
Video/OSCE-type alternatives (Leicester system)			
Trainers report			
MCQ			
Paperwork			

	CRS1 (date)	**CRS2** (date)	**CRS3** (date)

MRCGP
Pros/cons of sitting
Modules: Video
            Paper 1
            Paper 2
            Viva
            Simulated surgery			

Notes on use:

Trainer/facilitator-based methods

Manchester rating scales

This is Occasional Paper 40 published by the RCGP. Many trainers found sections of this useful to help define a problem, e.g. history taking appears to be a problem – scales 1 and 2 break this down into 10 constituent parts that may help identify where the problem lies. The scales cover:

- history taking
- physical examination
- problem definition
- management
- medical records
- emergency care
- professionalism
- personal development.

Copies can be obtained from: Central Sales Office, RCGP, 14 Princes Gate, London SW7 1PU (Tel: 020 7581 3232).

MCQ-based methods

- Phased evaluation programme (PEP) MCQs can be obtained from the College (see above) or downloaded from the College website on http:\\www.rcgp.org.com
- MCQ master can be obtained from Dr A Riaz, University of Birmingham, Dept of General Practice, Edgbaston, Birmingham B15 2TT (Tel: 0121 414 3763) (approximately £30).

Skills assessments

Self-awareness needs assessment

- ▶ Self-perception inventory: Belbin's team style questionnaire is available commercially from the London Video arts collection ISBN 0906807701 produced by J Hemingway and called 'Building the perfect team'.
- ▶ Learning styles questionnaire ⎫
- ▶ Influencing styles questionnaire ⎪
- ▶ Win–win questionnaire ⎬ all of these are available from Peter Honey, Ardingly House, 10 Linden Avenue, Maidenhead, Berks SL6 6HB (Tel: 01628 633946; Fax: 01628 633262)
- ▶ Counselling style questionnaire ⎪
- ▶ Interpersonal styles questionnaire ⎭
- ▶ Firo B 16 PF personality inventory was developed by Schutz and is published in *The Interpersonal World* by Science Behaviour Books, Palo Alto, CA, USA (available from Oxford Psychologists Press Ltd, Lambourne House, 311–321 Banbury Road, Oxford OX2 7JH; Tel: 01865 404500).
- ▶ *Crown Crisp Experiential Index* by A Crisp from Hodder and Stoughton.

Skills checklist

This is a specifically skills-related checklist that highlights areas for revisiting from the past and areas for development.

Skills I – Basics
This is the chance for the registrar to review the basic skills taught at medical school in order to identify any blindspots.

Tick all those you feel sufficiently confident about and highlight any you feel might need attention:

Palpation:	*Examination of:*
Apex beat	Neonate
Neck and thyroid	Children
Abdomen	Fractious children
Pulses	Pregnant women
Breast	Joints and spine
Percussion:	Eye: internal
Chest	external
Abdomen	Ears
Auscultation	Nose
Cardiac	Mouth
Respiratory	
Abdomen	Doing a PR exam
	Doing a VE exam
Others:	Passing a speculum PV: Simms
Script writing	Cusco
Note keeping	

Skills II – Essentials

These are the skills every GP should possess. Tick those you feel confident about and highlight those you would like to develop:

Swabs/urinanalysis:	*Resuscitation:*
Pernasal swab	Basic resuscitation
Cervical swab	(ABC) (including
Skin swab	mouth-to-mouth
MSU (including	and ECM)
techniques in children)	Heimlich manoeuvre
	IV infusion technique
	Basic first aid

Injections:
IV
IM
SC
ID
Venepuncture
Insulin injection

Minor surgery:
Antiseptic technique
Suturing
Incision of abscesses
Dressing principles
Ear syringing
Use of cautery/cryocautery
Use of curette
Draining of subungual haematoma
Local anaesthesia techniques
Foreign body removal: ear
                              eye
                              nose

Other:
Enemas
ECG interpretation
Spirometry interpretation
Audiometry interpretation
Tympanometry
   interpretation
Urinary catheterisation
Use of sonicaid
Proctoscope

Skills III – Special skills

A significant number of GPs have these skills but by no means all. Tick those you may have acquired and are confident about. Highlight those you would like to acquire:

Minor surgery:
Toenail surgery
Varicose vein surgery
Haemorrhoid surgery
Joint injection and aspiration
Skin biopsy
Aural toilet

Use of:
Microscope
Arterial doppler
Colposcope
Endoscope
Sigmoidoscope
Laryngoscope

Nasal packing	Tonometer
Excision of skin lesions	ESR apparatus
Hormonal implants	Haemoglobinometer
Norplant insertion	Clinical cameras
IUCD fitting	
Cap fitting	

The list of special skills many GPs possess is growing year by year.

Myers–Briggs type indicator – key elements

This indicator allows the trainer and learner to look at the effect of their own styles. It encourages self-awareness and an awareness of the variety and strengths of alternative styles. This table lists the key elements of each style and can be used for analysis and discussion.

Energising

Extrovert	*Introvert*
External – outside push	Internal – inside pull
Blurt it out	Keep it in
Breadth	Depth
People, things	Ideas, thoughts
Interaction	Concentration
Action	Reflection
Do–think–do	Think–do–think

Attending

Sensing	*Intuiting*
The five senses	Sixth sense
What is real	What could be
Practical	Theoretical/heretical
Present	Future
Facts	Meanings/insights
Using established skills	Looking for new skills

Practicality	Novelty
Step by step	Leaps and bounds

Deciding

Thinking	*Feeling*
Head	Heart
Logical	Comfortable
Objective	Subjective
Justice	Mercy
Critique	Compliment
Principles	Harmony
Reason	Empathy
Firm and fair	Compassion

Living

Judging	*Perceiving*
Plans	Spontaneous
Regulates	Flows
Controls	Adapts
Settled	Tentative
Control the system	See what happens
Set goals	Head in directions
Decisive	Open
Organised	Flexible

Thinking styles I

An appreciation of your own thinking style and that of the person you are communicating with improves the interaction. This is a simple model that can be used for discussion:

> ▸ The DREAMER forms new goals and ideas without the fetters of reality
> ▸ The REALIST tries to convert the dream into possible expression
> ▸ The CRITIC/EVALUATOR refines and checks the process

The DREAMER asks   – What do we want to do?
  – When do we want to
    do it?
  – What do we hope to gain
    from doing it?

'anything is possible'

The REALIST asks   – How can we do it?
  – Who will do it?
  – Where will we do it?
  – When will we do it?

'some things are possible'

The CRITIC/EVALUATOR asks
  – What effect will this have?
  – Who will it effect?
  – What could stop it?

'not everything is possible'

Questions for registrar and trainer:

► Where do you fit into this spectrum?
► What effect does this have?
► Is the model useful in any other context?
► Can you identify other members of the PHCT or patients
  where this would have helped manage a situation?

Personality style inventory

This identifies the primary style the user applies when
interacting with other people or new situations. It allows
discussion of the advantages/disadvantages of the style
and raises the question of trying to experiment with other
styles.

Instructions
Look at the following pairs of words and ask which of
them most typifies your behaviour. Tick A if you strongly

identify with the word on the left, tick B if less so, C if you identify more with the word on the right and D if you strongly identify with the right-hand word.

A B C D	
Talks to	Listens to
Action	Reaction
Going step by step	Getting whole picture
Quick paced	Deliberate
Experimenting	Digesting
Carrying out ideas	Thinking up ideas
Working for change	Working for stability
Animated	Reserved
Doing	Watching
Finding solutions	Identifying problems
Answering questions	Asking questions
Improvising	Planning
Pragmatic	Idealistic
Concerned with the end	Concerned with the means

Do the same with the following using the 1–4 scale:

	1 2 3 4	
Intuition		Logic
Personal		Impersonal
Emotional		Intellectual
Having an opinion		Having a conceptual model
Discuss with others		Analyse oneself
Look for new experiences		Look for new ideas
Accepting		Questioning
Feeling		Thinking
Takes risks		Calculates
Trial and error		Plan and organise
People-orientated		Task-orientated
Gets involved		Looks for faults
Seeks out others		Works alone
Gives support		Gives a critique

Count the ticks in each column and circle the highest score for A to D and 1 to 4. Plot them on the scale below by following these three steps:

1 draw a line down the boxes starting from your high score letter
2 draw a line across starting from your high score number
3 put a cross where the lines intersect.

That's your style!

```
                        FEELER
            A      B       C       D
    1     ENTHUSIASTIC    IMAGINATIVE    I
      D                                  N
    2                                    T
      O                                  U
    3                                    I
      E    PRACTICAL        LOGICAL      T
    4                                    E
      R              THINKER             R
```

If you have ties you may have two primary styles (or think you have). If you tie between B and D then you are probably C. If you score in the corners (A1, D1, A4 or D4) then you strongly identify with the style.

Now look at the next two sections.

SUMMARY OF PERSONALITY TYPE DESCRIPTIONS

Enthusiastic
- feeling and doing
- rushes in on trial and error 'gut' feeling
- seeks others' opinions and feelings for support
- likes risk and challenge
- thrives on new situations
- impulsive
- emotional
- looks forward

Imaginative
- feeling and intuiting
- sees whole picture and options
- uses imagination
- bursts of energy
- uses insight
- unhurried, casual, friendly
- listens, observes
- likes assurance of others

Practical
- doing and thinking
- applies ideas and theories
- searches and solves thoughtfully
- likes control
- acts independently and then looks for feedback
- learns by testing out

Logical
- feeling and thinking
- uses models and theories in thinking
- brings things together slowly and thoughtfully
- uses past experience
- organised, precise and analytical
- avoids over-emotion

These summaries can be used as a basis for discussion.

ADVANTAGES AND DISADVANTAGES OF PERSONALITY TYPES

Enthusiast

Advantages
- takes risks
- gets involved and involves others
- wants ideas and options from everyone
- uses gut reaction

Disadvantages
- disorganised and no goals set
- impulsive
- changing
- demanding
- overcommits

Imaginative

- many creative ideas
- can wait for correct time
- sees perspective
- sensitive to others/stresses

- waits too long
- can't see the trees for the wood
- uncritical
- all ideas and no action
- frustrating to others

Practical	**Logical**
Advantages	
– evaluates and sets goals works well alone	– gathers facts and is organised
– likes problem solving	– reviews and calculates
– likes action	– works well alone
	– uses past experience
Disadvantages	
– reckless and impatient in action	– obsessed with gathering evidence
– undervalues personal feelings	– undervalues all feelings and fails to recognise stress
– tends to overcontrol	– overcautious
– underuses others	– overinfluenced by past

Miller–Smith lifestyle assessment inventory

This is a stress awareness tool and might be useful if the registrar has a problem in this area or even just as a tool to generate interest in a tutorial on burnout and stress.

Instructions
Read each item carefully and give it a rating of 1 to 5 according to the scale below:

1 = almost always
2 = often
3 = sometimes
4 = occasionally
5 = almost never

1 I eat at least one hot, balanced meal a day
2 I give and receive affection regularly
3 I get 7–8 hours sleep per night at least four days a week

4 I have a living relative within 30 miles on whom I can rely

5 I exercise to the point of perspiration at least twice a week

6 I smoke fewer than 10 cigarettes per day

7 I drink fewer than five drinks per week

8 I am the appropriate weight for my height

9 I have an adequate income to meet my basic needs

10 I get strength from my religion *or* I am comfortable with my view of existence and my place in the world

11 I regularly attend social activities

12 I have a network of friends and acquaintances

13 I have at least one friend to confide in with regard to personal matters

14 I am in good health

15 I am able to speak openly about my feelings

16 I have regular conversations with the people I live with about daily living issues

17 I do something for fun at least once a week.

18 I am able to organise my time effectively

19 I drink fewer than three cups of coffee (or tea/cocoa) per day

20 I take a quiet time for myself daily

Add the scores and interpret them as below. The range is 20–100.

- ► 30–40 is about expected.
- ► 40–50 suggests it is time to take stock and look at stress reduction techniques.
- ► 50–60 suggests a real problem.
- ► 60+ should have everyone hearing alarm bells.

By looking at the high-score items the scale can be used to suggest some stress reduction strategies.

Assertiveness rights questionnaire

This is a questionnaire that gives the user some insight into their assertiveness skills.

Instructions
Look at the statements below and mark each one against the scale provided:

	Strongly agree	Agree	Neutral	Disagree	Strongly disagree
▶ I have the right to set my own priorities					
▶ I have the right to tell others what I am feeling					
▶ I have the right to be heard					
▶ I have the right to require an explanation of others actions if they affect me					
▶ I have the right to say no without explanation					
▶ I have the right to insist that I get what I pay for					
▶ I have the right to break with convention if I wish to					
▶ I have the right to make mistakes without feeling guilty					
▶ I have the right to express myself if I wish					
▶ I have the right to spend some time each day as I wish					
▶ I have the right to my own physical space					
▶ I have the right to ask for what I want					

Add up the total of ticks in each vertical column and score them as below:

Strongly agree   ticks × 5
Agree   × 4
Neutral   × 3
Disagree   × 2
Strongly disagree   × 1

_____

Overall total

_____

Score significance:

>45:   you are basically assertive

30–45: you are variable in your approach; is it certain situations or people that influence you? Look at your low scoring areas to help identify these

<30:   you are unlikely to be assertive and need to reflect on the attitudes that underpin your response.

Other aspects of this scale and assertiveness are covered in the section in Chapter 6 on team skills.

Motivating values scale

This is a simple rank ordering scale that allows analysis and provokes discussion about motivation. It can help both the registrar and trainer understand the drivers at work. It is often helpful for the trainer to do the exercise too.

Place the following words in a rank order (with the most important at the top) that reflects how important you feel these concepts are in your life.

Independence – freedom to do what you believe is best

Power – to feel in control of your situation

Self-fulfilment – to be able to enjoy your potential

Duty – doing what is expected of you

Nurturing – looking after others

Friendship – being liked and having companions

Family – meeting the needs of your family

Wealth – earning a lot of money

Pleasure – being happy and having fun

Expertness – being the best at something

Leadership – having and influencing followers

Health – taking care of yourself

Security – having no worries about income or welfare

Self-awareness summary sheet – the initial assessment grid

This is a form designed to pull all the needs assessment areas together. It contains fields to record the assessments of knowledge, confidence rating scales (CRS), record the past experience and to put in a process related 'gut' score if desired. When completed it highlights areas for more detailed consideration.

Subject area	Experience[1]	PEP score[2]	CRS score[3]	Practice score[4]
General surgery				
Orthopaedics				
Urology				
Casualty				
General medicine				
Paediatrics				
Therapeutics				
Rheumatology				

Dermatology
ENT
Ophthalmology

Obstetrics
Gynaecology
Family planning

General practice
Consultation skills
Management
Finances
Education
Self-awareness

Anaesthetics

Minor surgery

Audit

Preventative care

[1]Record months in hospital posts, examinations, courses, etc.
[2]PEP score from MCQ
[3]CRS score 1–5
[4]Practice score 1–5
1 = poor, 2 = below average, 3 = average , 4 = above average,
5 = excellent
CRS = confidence rating scales.

Assessment of attitudinal needs

This is usually a process-related assessment although the following form was offered as a way of assessing attitudes.

It is an analogue scale tool where you allocate a mark on the line between two extreme statements:

1 The registrar is —————— The registrar does
   caring and   not seem to care
   compassionate   or show compassion

2 The registrar is —————— The registrar is
   conscientious in   slapdash in
   approach   approach

3 The registrar is —————— The registrar is
   punctual   often late

4 The registrar is —————— The registrar is
   interested and   disinterested and
   enthusiastic   bored

5 The registrar is —————— The registrar is
   approachable   unreceptive/
   and friendly   unresponsive

6 The registrar has —————— The registrar seems
   good relationships   isolated
   in and outside of
   the practice

7 The registrar —————— The registrar is
   seems to recognise   intolerant of any
   and respect the   views but their own
   values of others

8 The registrar has ———————— The registrar
a positive attitude appears to resent
to teaching the educational
and learning process

It can help to identify attitudinal problem areas for discussion.

The other approach was to use ethical scenarios to generate discussion which would have a value laden content. A few suggestions are described below.

Example 1
Ask the registrar to find some recent newspaper cuttings demonstrating some medical ethical conflicts (there are always some) and use these as a basis for discussion.

Example 2
Ask the registrar to note the next five consultations where they became aware of an ethical dilemma. The trainer can also bring their next five.

Example 3
A patient you know well has cancelled his holiday because his car broke down and he needed the money. He asks you to fill in an insurance form to say he was too ill to go – he says he had a 'virus' but didn't see a doctor.

Example 4
A 13-year-old girl is pregnant – she consults with her 17-year-old boyfriend. They want you to arrange a termination but say you mustn't tell her parents (try making the boyfriend 40 years old).

Example 5
A 25-year-old Asian lady with limited English language skills comes with her mother-in-law as interpreter. She

had symptoms of a PV loss and has now returned for the swab results, which show chlamydia.

Example 6

A man angrily tells you how his son was recently admitted with appendicitis. A partner saw him earlier on the day of admission and said he had a 'tummy bug'. The man says 'the surgeon said he almost had peritonitis and really should have been admitted earlier'.

Example 7

Mrs Jones is on long-term medication. She says 'I can't afford the prescription fees – can you give me 6 months medication at a time? I won't waste it'.

Example 8

Ask the registrar to do a 'personal construct analysis' of the ethical situations they find most challenging.

The list of 'virtual' patients is potentially endless and it is undoubtedly better to try and draw out the same points based on the registrar's own patients.

Other needs assessment methods

20-note review form

This is a format suggested for structured note reviews. Reviewing 20 notes in this way takes about 10–15 minutes and generates a number of learning needs. It is really case analysis without the registrar and, despite its obvious limitations, expands the trainer's knowledge of the registrar's behaviour with little time or effort expenditure.

Note identifier (no.)	Diagnosis comment	Prescribing comment	Records comment	Notes

The trainer must be careful to restrict himself or herself to observations, as the notes are out of the consultation context. However, many trainers find this process a good source of material for discussion. It can be 'programmed' on a regular basis (e.g. as a 3-monthly exercise).

Personal construct analysis
This technique is described in the text but further details can be found in a paper by Dunn (1993) 'Personal construct analysis – a teaching tool for trainers'. The registrar basically produces a list of 10 points on a particular theme. It is easily adapted to allow the registrar to drive the educational agenda, e.g. do a list for what they find the 10 most difficult presentations. It can be used to bring out attitudes, e.g. list the 10 characteristics of difficult patients.

Registrar 'wish' list
This is a simple form that asks the registrar to declare his or her own agenda.

THE REGISTRAR WISH LIST – or what do I want to achieve in my training period?

Keep it simple, i.e. a maximum of six in each column. They don't have to be medical at all!

Knowledge (areas to expand)	Skills (practicalities)	Attitudes (how you will feel or think)	Personal (anything)	Other (anything else)

Staff feedback – the Abbotswood forms
Many practices mentioned the use of feedback from staff in assessing needs. This seems an underused approach with great potential. The Abbotswood practice has formalised this and some of their forms are shown.

ABBOTTSWOOD MEDICAL CENTRE

RECEPTION EVALUATION OF GP REGISTRAR

REGISTRAR: .... DATE: ....

	Very good	Good	Average	Poor	Very poor
	1	2	3	4	5

1 Communication

2 Attitude to staff

3 Patient response

4 Running to time
  in surgery

5 Flexibility

6 Personality

Comments ....
....
....
....
....

ABBOTTSWOOD MEDICAL CENTRE

PRACTICE MANAGER EVALUATION OF GP REGISTRAR

REGISTRAR: .... DATE: ....

Very good / Good / Average / Poor / Very poor
1   2   3   4   5

1 Attitude to staff

2 Reasonable
holiday leave and
study leave requests

3 Interest in
management issues

4 Understanding of
management issues

5 Personality

6 Displays
responsibility for
self e.g. personal
accounts/admin, etc.

Comments ....
....
....
....
....

ABBOTTSWOOD MEDICAL CENTRE

PRACTICE NURSE EVALUATION OF
GP REGISTRAR

REGISTRAR: .... DATE: ....

Very good / Good / Average / Poor / Very poor
  1   2   3   4   5

1 Accessibility

2 Approachability

3 Attitude to staff/
   patients

4 Commitment to
   patient care

5 Communication
   with staff and
   patients

6 Is he/she receptive
   to requests from
   nursing staff
   regarding
   information and/
   or patient needs?

Comments ....
....
....
....
....

ABBOTTSWOOD MEDICAL CENTRE

**DISTRICT NURSES EVALUATION OF
GP REGISTRAR**

REGISTRAR: .... DATE: ....

Very good / Good / Average / Poor / Very poor
1　　　　2　　　　3　　　　4　　　　5

1 Appropriate
referrals

2 Attitude to district
nursing staff

3 Access to
GP registrar

4 Communication
liaison

Comments ....

....

....

....

....

► REFERENCES

Al-Shehri A (1995) Learning by reflection. *Education for General Practice.* 7: 237–48.

Balint M (1957) *The Doctor, His Patient and the Illness.* Pitman Medical, London.

Balint E and Norell J (1973) *Six Minutes for the Patient.* Tavistock, London.

Barrington (1985) *The Hemispheric Mode Indicator: right and left brain approaches to learning.* Excel.

Barrow H and Tamblyn R (1980) *Problem Based Learning: an approach to medical training.* Springer.

Battles J *et al.* (1990) The affective attributes of the ideal primary care specialist. In: W Bender *et al.* (eds) *Teaching and Assessing Clinical Competence.* Boek Werk.

Belbin R (1981) *Management Teams: why they succeed or fail.* Heinemann, Oxford.

Berne E (1977) *Games People Play.* Penguin, Harmondsworth.

Blanchard K (1982) *Leadership and the One Minute Manager.* Blanchard Management Press, London.

Bligh J (1992) Independent learning among GP trainees: an initial survey. *Medical Education.* **26**: 497–50.

Bligh J (1993) The S-SDRLS: a short questionnaire about self directed learning. *Education for General Practice.* **4**: 121–5.

Brown G and Atkins M (1988) *Effective Teaching in Higher Education.* Methuen, London.

Burnard P (1991) *Teaching Interpersonal Skills.* Chapman and Hall, London.

Byrne B and Long P (1976) *Doctors Talking to Patients.* HMSO, London.

Campion P *et al.* (1997) *Teaching Medicine in the Community.* Oxford Medical GP Series, Oxford.

Coulson R and Osbourne C (1984) Ensuring curricular content in a student directed problem based learning programme. In: H Schmidt and M De Volder (eds) *Tutorials in Problem Based Learning.* Van Gorcum.

Cox K and Ewan C (1988) *The Medical Teacher.* Churchill Livingstone, Edinburgh.

Department of Health (2000) *The GP Registrar Scheme: vocational training for general medical practice. The UK guide.* DoH, London.

Dunn A (1993) Personal construct analysis. *Education for General Practice.* **2**: 121–5.

Fabb W (1997) WONCA. Proceedings of the Educational Symposium.

Fabb W *et al.* (1976) *Focus on Learning.* RACGP Family Medicine Programme. Beavergroup, Melbourne.

Foulkes F and Fulton P (1991) Critical appraisal of published literature. *BMJ.* **302**: 1136.

Freeling P and Browne K (1976) *The Doctor–Patient Relationship.* Churchill Livingstone, New York.

Fry J (1972) *The Future General Practitioner.* RCGP, London.

Glasser W (1965) *Reality Therapy.* Harper and Row, London.

Guilbert J (1997) *Education Handbook for Health Personnel.* Offset Publication No. 35, WHO, Geneva.

Hall D (1983) *A GP Trainer's Handbook.* Blackwell Scientific Press, Oxford.

Harden R *et al.* (1998) The continuum of problem based learning. *Medical Teacher.* **20**: 317.

Harris T (1973) *I'm OK, You're OK.* Pan Books, London.

Havelock P *et al.* (1997) *Professional Education for General Practice.* Oxford Medical GP Series, Oxford.

Helman D (1981) Disease versus illness in general practice. *JRCGP.* **31**: 548–53.

Helman C (1984) *JRCGP.* **34**: 547–50.

Heron J (1986) *Six Category Intervention Analysis: human potential research project.* University of Surrey, Guildford.

Hewson P and Gollan R (1995) *Journal of Paediatrics and Child Health.* **31**: 29–32.

Honey P and Mumford A (1992) *The Manual of Learning Styles.* Peter Honey, Maidenhead.

Howard J (1997) The emotional diary: a framework for reflective learning. *Education for General Practice.* **8**: 288–91.

Irby D (1992) *Academic Medicine.* **67**(10): 630–8.

ICGP (1991) Time management: key ideas. In: *Handbook and Diary.* ICGP, Dublin.

JCGPT (1992) *Training for General Practice.* JCGPT, London.

JCGPT (1992) *Accreditation of Regions and Schemes for Vocational Training in General Practice: general guidance.* JCGPT, London.

JCPTGP (2000) *Recommendations to Regions for Establishment Criteria for the Approval and Re-approval of Trainers in General Practice.* JCPTGP, London.

Jensen E (1994) *Superteaching: turning points for teachers.* Barron's Educational Series.

Knowles M (1973) *Self Directed Learning: a guide for teachers and learners.* Association Press.

Kolb D (1974) *Experiential Learning.* Prentice Hall, London.

Kurtz S, Silverman J and Draper J (1998) *Teaching and Learning Communication Skills in Medicine.* Radcliffe Medical Press, Oxford.

Landsberg M (1997) *The Tao of Coaching.* Knowledge Exchange, Santa Monica, CA.

Levenstein J *et al.* (1986) *Family Practice.* **3**(1): 24–30.

Lublin J (1992) Role modelling: a case study in GP. *Medical Education.* **26**: 116–22.

Macauley D (1994) READER: an acronym for critical appraisal. *BJGP.* **44**: 83–5.

McWhinney I (1972) Problem solving and decision making in primary medical practice. *Proceedings of the Royal Society of Medicine.* **65**(11): 934–8.

Maslow A (1972) *Motivation and Personality.* Harper and Row, New York.

Matthews P, Skelton J, Wiskin C and Field S (1999) *Sex-lives and Videotape: sexual history taking in primary care.* Radcliffe Medical Press, Oxford.

McEvoy P (1998) *Educating the Future GP* (2e). Radcliffe Medical Press, Oxford.

Miller *et al.* (1998) Motivation to learn. *BJGP.* **48**: 1429–32.

Murtagh J (1998) *General Practice.* McGraw Hill, London.

Myerscough P and Ford J (1996) *Talking with Patients.* Oxford Medical GP Series, Oxford.

Neame L (1984) Problem orientated learning in medical education. In: H Schmidt and M De Volder (eds) *Tutorials in Problem Based Learning.* Van Goeren.

Neighbour R (1987) *The Inner Consultation.* Kluwer Academic.

Neighbour R (1992) *The Inner Apprentice.* Kluwer Academic.

O'Connor J (1993) *An Introduction to NLP.* Aquarian Press, San Francisco, CA.

Pendleton D, Schofield T, Havelock P and Tate P (1984) *The Consultation: an approach to learning and teaching.* Oxford Medical GP Series, Oxford.

Pereira Gray D (1979) *A system of training for general practice.* Occasional paper 4. RCGP, London.

Pitts J (1996) Pathologies of 1:1 teaching. *Education for General Practice.* **7**: 118–22.

Prochaska SO and DiClemente CL (1986) Towards a comprehensive model of change. In: WR Miller and N Heather (eds) *Treating Addictive Behaviours: processes of change*. Plenum Press.

Quirk M (1994) *How to Learn and Teach in Medical School*. Charles C Thomas.

RCGP (1988) *Priority objectives for general practice vocational training*. Occasional paper 30. RCGP, London.

RCGP (1989) *Rating scales for vocational training in general practice*. Occasional paper 40. RCGP, London.

Riding R and Cheema I (1991) Cognitive styles: an overview and integration. *Educational Psychology*. **11**: 193–215.

Rose C (1985) *Accelerated Learning*. Topaz.

Ruscoe M (1994) Assessment of the tutorial. *Education for General Practice*. **5**: 260–8.

Sandars J and Baron R (1988) *Learning GP: a structured approach*. Pastest Books, Hemel Hempstead.

Schon D (1987) *Educating the Reflective Practitioner: towards a new design for teaching and learning in the professions*. Jossey-Bass, Oxford.

Seedhouse D (1992) Avoiding the myths: a pre-requisite for teaching ethics. *Education for General Practice*. **3**: 117–24.

Shrebeneck P (1994) *The Death of Humane Medicine and the Rise of Coercive Healthism*. Social Affairs Unit, London.

Silverman J, Draper J and Kurtz S (1998) *Skills for Communicating with Patients*. Radcliffe Medical Press, Oxford.

Skelton J, Field S, Wiskin C and Tate P (1998) *Those Things You Say ...: consultation skills and the MRCGP examination*. Radcliffe Medical Press, Oxford.

Skelton J, Field S, Hammond P and Wiskin C (1999) *Watching You, Watching Me: consultation skills and summative assessment in general practice* (2e). Radcliffe Medical Press, Oxford.

Stewart M and Lieberman J (1993) *The 15 Minute Hour: applied psychotherapy for the primary care physician.* Praegar.

Stott N and Davis R (1979) The exceptional potential in each primary care consultation. *JRCGP.* **66**: 201–5.

Strasser R (1991) How we teach key aspects of general practice. *Medical Teacher.* **1**: 93.

Tate P (1998) *The Doctor's Communication Handbook* (2e). Radcliffe Medical Press, Oxford.

Tudor-Hart J (1989) *A New Kind of Doctor.* Merlin, London.

Turner J *et al.* (1998) Assessment of trainer performance in RCA. *Education for General Practice.* **9**: 199–202.

▶ INDEX